The Secrets to Sensational
FOREPLAY

The Secrets to Sensational FOREPLAY

THE HOTTEST WAY TO TOUCH YOUR LOVER FOR INCREDIBLE PLEASURE,
STRONGER ORGASMS, AND LONGER, BETTER SEX

LAURA ROSS

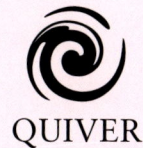

QUIVER

Text © 2011 Laura Ross
Photography © 2011 Quiver

First published in the USA in 2011 by
Quiver, a member of
Quayside Publishing Group
100 Cummings Center
Suite 406-L
Beverly, MA 01915-6101
www.quiverbooks.com

The Publisher maintains the records relating to images in this book required by 18 USC 2257. Records are located at Rockport Publishers, Inc., 100 Cummings Center, Suite 406-L, Beverly, MA 01915-6101.

15 14 13 12 11   1 2 3 4 5

ISBN-13: 978-1-59233-428-5
ISBN-10: 1-59233-428-8

Library of Congress Cataloging-in-Publication Data available

Photography: Holly Randall
Additional Photography: Lucua Scarlatti, page 7, 81, 84, 87, 90, 93, 98, 114,
                        117, 134, 145, 147, 155
                        Alan Penn, page 140

Printed and bound in Singapore

Dedication

For LBZ, who knows how to make a first date last for a decade.

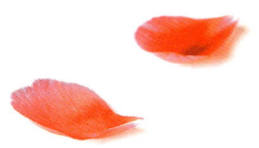

CONTENTS

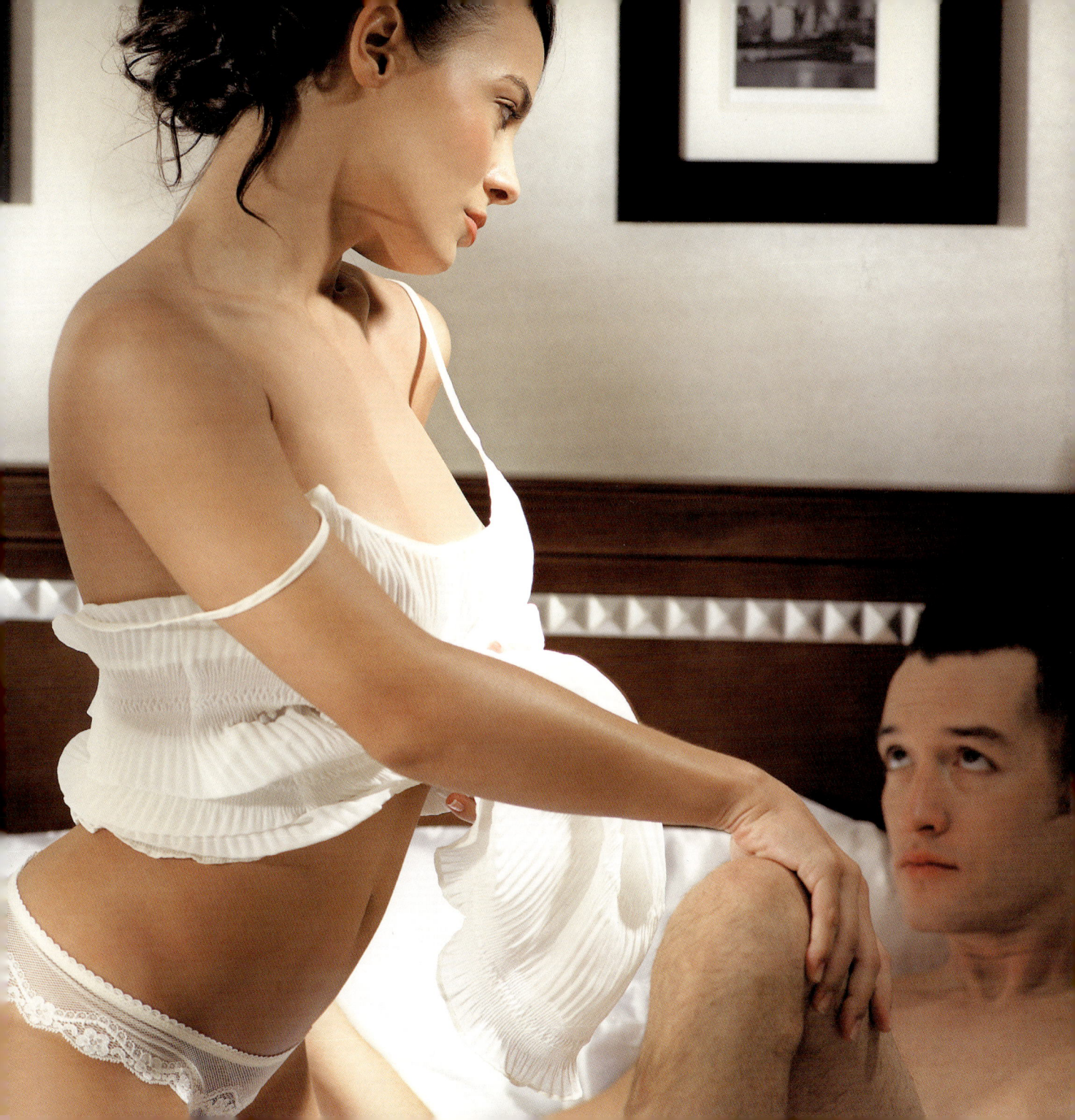

INTRODUCTION

Foreplay is like a thrilling journey undertaken with no map, no itinerary, no particular destination, and no arrival time. It is all about improvising, responding to each other, staying in tune, and sharing.

Many people view foreplay as a means for getting in the mood. That much is true. But here's something you may not know: Great foreplay can make great sex even better! Foreplay doesn't just rev up your engine—it can make each delicious moment of sex more pleasurable and rewarding. What's more, good foreplay can actually make orgasms much more intense for both of you. All that teasing, kissing, fondling, and stroking (and maybe even role-playing, fantasizing, "sexting," or other preliminaries) help send the blood rushing to your nipples, your clitoris or your cock . . . heightening the sensitivity . . . so when you do reach that climax—fireworks. Talented lovers the world over know that sizzling foreplay leads to super-hot sex—and sex experts know that that can lead to a fulfilling relationship in the bedroom and beyond.

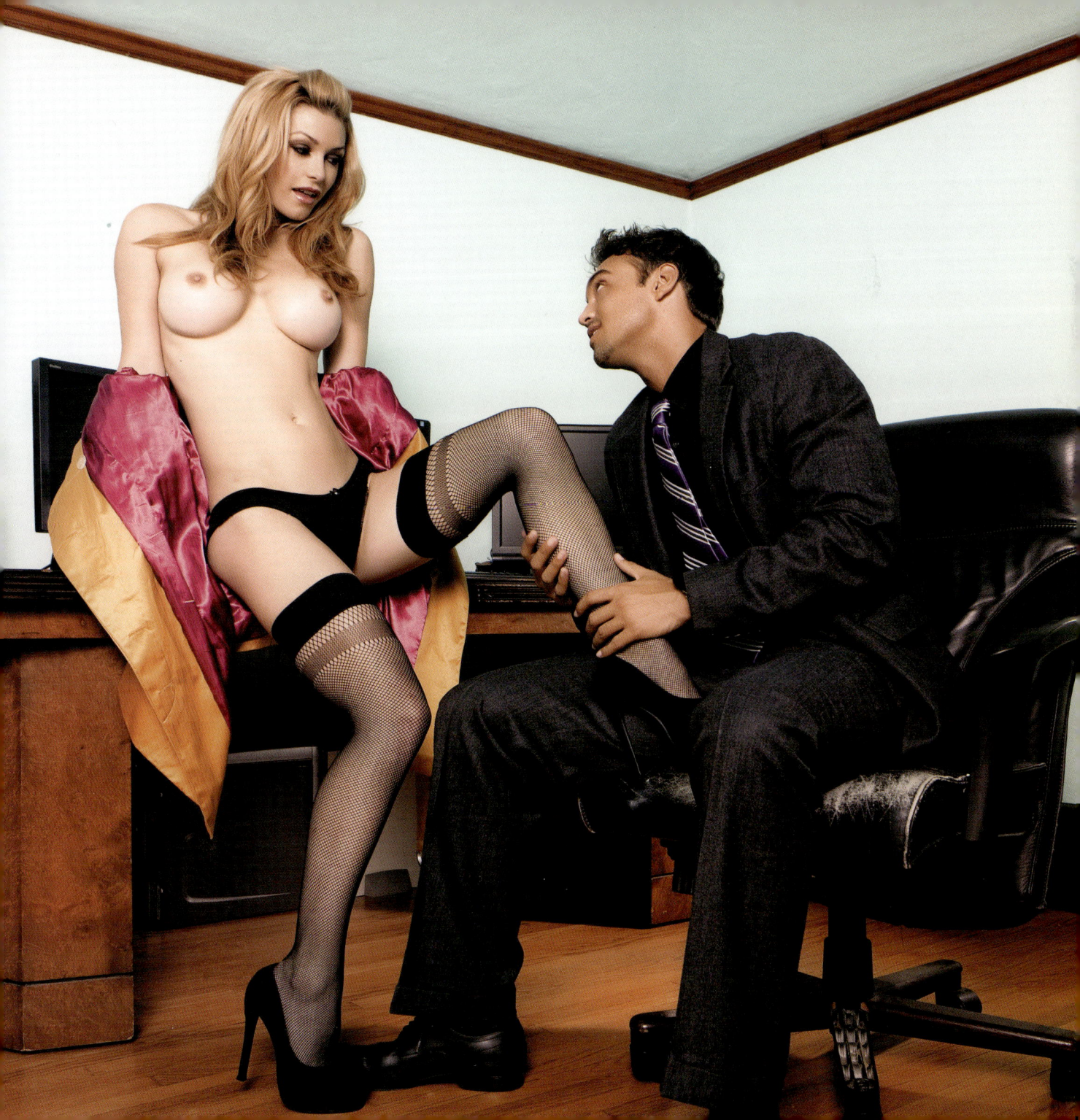

*M*aybe you are already pretty adept in the foreplay department, but wonder what new tricks you might try. Or perhaps you and your mate would like to understand one another's needs a little bit better by getting the 4-1-1 from an expert. Whatever your reasons for being here, welcome to *better, sexier sex.*

Here's another little-known fact: There's more to an exciting sex life than penetration and orgasm. The real sexual hero isn't the one with the most generous endowment, the longest-lasting erection, or the proclivity for multiple orgasms (though we *all* have that potential hidden inside of us, dying to come out). It's the person with the wildest imagination, the deepest responsiveness, and the most care for his or her partner; it's the person who involves the whole body as well as the mind in the act of lovemaking and who takes the time to enjoy it all to the fullest. With some thought—and the guidance and inspiration of this book—you and your partner can reach new heights of pleasure and mutual understanding. You've already taken the first step. Now all you have to do is open your mind to this new adventure and the sky is the limit for pleasure for both of you.

I'd like to do away with one huge myth right off the bat: Men don't want or need foreplay, but women do. In fact, plenty of studies show that men need and want foreplay just as much as women do. And even if they don't *know* they want a warm-up, once they've experienced some luxurious, inspired foreplay, they may never again rush to the main event. That's why this book offers lots of tips, tricks, and techniques specific to each gender. (For techniques that can be employed by both of you, I switch up the pronouns randomly—e.g., "stroke *her* leg"; "nibble *his* earlobe.")

Of course there are physiological differences between the genders. If you want to get technical, studies show that women need at least fifteen minutes of concentrated foreplay for the purposes of lubrication and expansion of the vaginal canal. As for men, let's just say that what they need physically and what they are capable of enjoying may be two different things. But regardless of what you need and how long it takes you to get ready, great foreplay is all about opening new doors to pleasure and involving all five of your senses.

The word *sensual* is sometimes used interchangeably with *sexual*. The two are certainly related, but *sensual* really refers to the five senses. Truly sensual foreplay involves waking up and heightening each one of these senses: sight, hearing, smell, taste, and touch. That last sense—touch—is the obvious suspect in foreplay (and much of this book is devoted to it), but don't discount the importance of the other senses in achieving the height of pleasure (along with that sixth one—intuition.). Expanding your foreplay vocabulary involves learning about sounds, from carefully selected music to moans of ecstasy; sights, from watching each other undress to sharing sexy movies; tastes, from aphrodisiac foods to your own salty skin; and smells, from perfumed light bulbs and bedsheets to the musky aroma of sex itself. The goal: learning to bring every one of your senses into play for a truly *sensual* sexual experience.

The first step on your sensual journey, covered in chapter 1, is flirtation and seduction. Great foreplay starts long before you reach the bedroom. By focusing on yourself, your clothing, your movements, even your words, you can create the tension of anticipation between you and your lover. Think of flirtation and seduction as a trail of teasing breadcrumbs leading to the pleasure dome; once you reach your destination, you can further draw out the anticipation of the pleasure to come by using any one—or all—of your senses and the techniques in this book.

Chapter 2 is all about the many ways you can use your mouth to drive your partner crazy. Kissing is just the beginning when you get oral; there are so many *kinds* of kisses, and so many other ways to use your mouths on each other, simultaneously and in turn. While this book doesn't include a detailed discussion of oral sex—because I feel it falls under the definition of *sex*, not foreplay—I have included a number of oral techniques that work well in the foreplay arena. On the other hand, I do talk about orgasms (having them as well as holding them back) because I believe they can be an integral part of foreplay—if you want them to be, that is.

Next, in chapter 3, you'll explore all of the ways you can use touch on your partner, from simple caresses, gentle fondling, or true manhandling to delicious all-over massage. Need a brushup on erogenous zones? You'll get a complete road map of your partner, from earlobe to pinky toe. Foreplay kicks into high gear when you let your fingers and hands do the walking.

In chapter 4, I offer up the promised land: the genitalia. Once you've breached the panty/boxer barrier, you're on the road to mutual ecstasy, and there are dozens of specific techniques you can use to heighten the experience—including deliciously satisfying masturbation. Forget what your mother told you: It's perfectly natural (alone or together) and H-O-T!

Taking on new personalities can be liberating, and pretending to be strangers can bring you closer together. chapter 5 introduces the luscious world of role-playing, where you can live out your fantasies and those of your lover, and discover each other all over again. Just to get you started, I've concocted some killer scenarios for you to try out together.

If you're ready to experience edgier foreplay, chapter 6 delves into the realm of rough play, sex toys, restraint, bondage, pornography, and other more daring sexual activities. Whether or not you think of yourselves as "edgy," there are plenty of ideas here for those nights when you and your partner are feeling a bit more adventurous than usual and are ready to explore all your fantasies.

Next, it's time to move beyond the bedroom. In chapter 7, you'll submerge yourself in the world of watery foreplay fun. Water is a great medium for sex play, whether you are in your own bathtub or shower, or in an outdoor pool or backyard hot tub.

Finally, I've included chapters about fun in public places, the not-so-subtle art of talking dirty, and more. And don't miss my Love Questionnaire, which is designed to help you and your partner communicate your deepest desires in positive language that will enhance your sex life rather than create barriers between you. It's a basic fact: You can't have transcendent sex without great communication.

Sublime foreplay is about imbuing everything you do with sexual energy—making the world a sexy place day and night, when you are together and even when you are apart. That fabulous glow you feel after great sex can last all day long. It can cement you together as a couple and fill you both with joy. The final section of this book is called "Afterplay" because the ultimate goal is to help you prolong the sensations of sex beyond the bedroom. Foreplay (and sex itself) is all about mutual understanding, openness, willingness to take risks within the trusting bond you've established, and reaching new heights of pleasure together.

Enjoy!

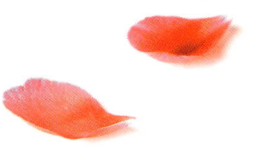

Part I:
Teaseplay

Flirtation, Seduction, and Red-Hot Romance

When do you think foreplay begins? When you step into the bedroom? When you take your clothes off? Dynamite foreplay—the kind that turns your lover into a pool of melted butter, responsive to your every whim—can (and should!) begin long before you enter the bedroom and fire up those luscious sensory techniques.

Foreplay begins with flirtation, proceeds through seduction, and has a lot to do with romance. And although it's true that not everyone you make eye contact with at a party will end up in your bed, making any potential partner ache with anticipation is the first leg of your sexual journey together, and a great way to set the tone for all that follows.

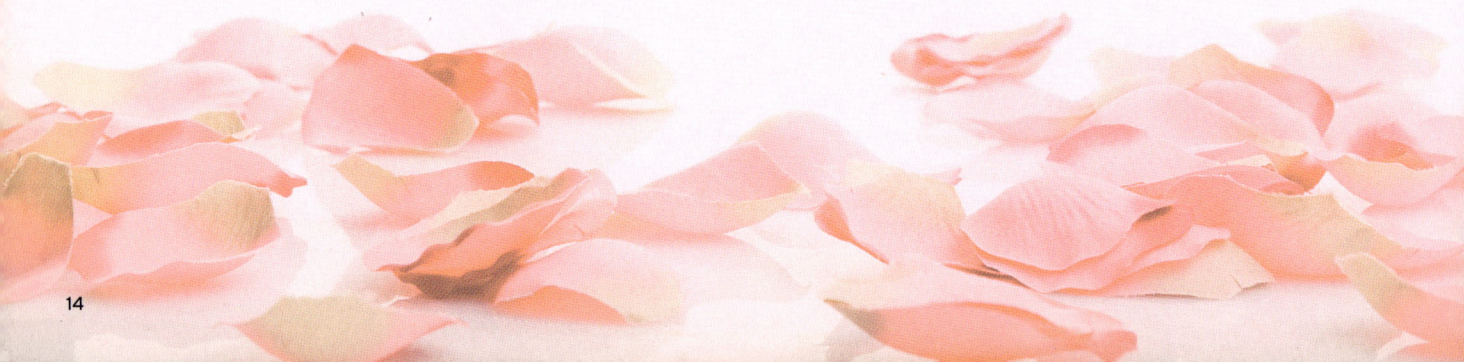

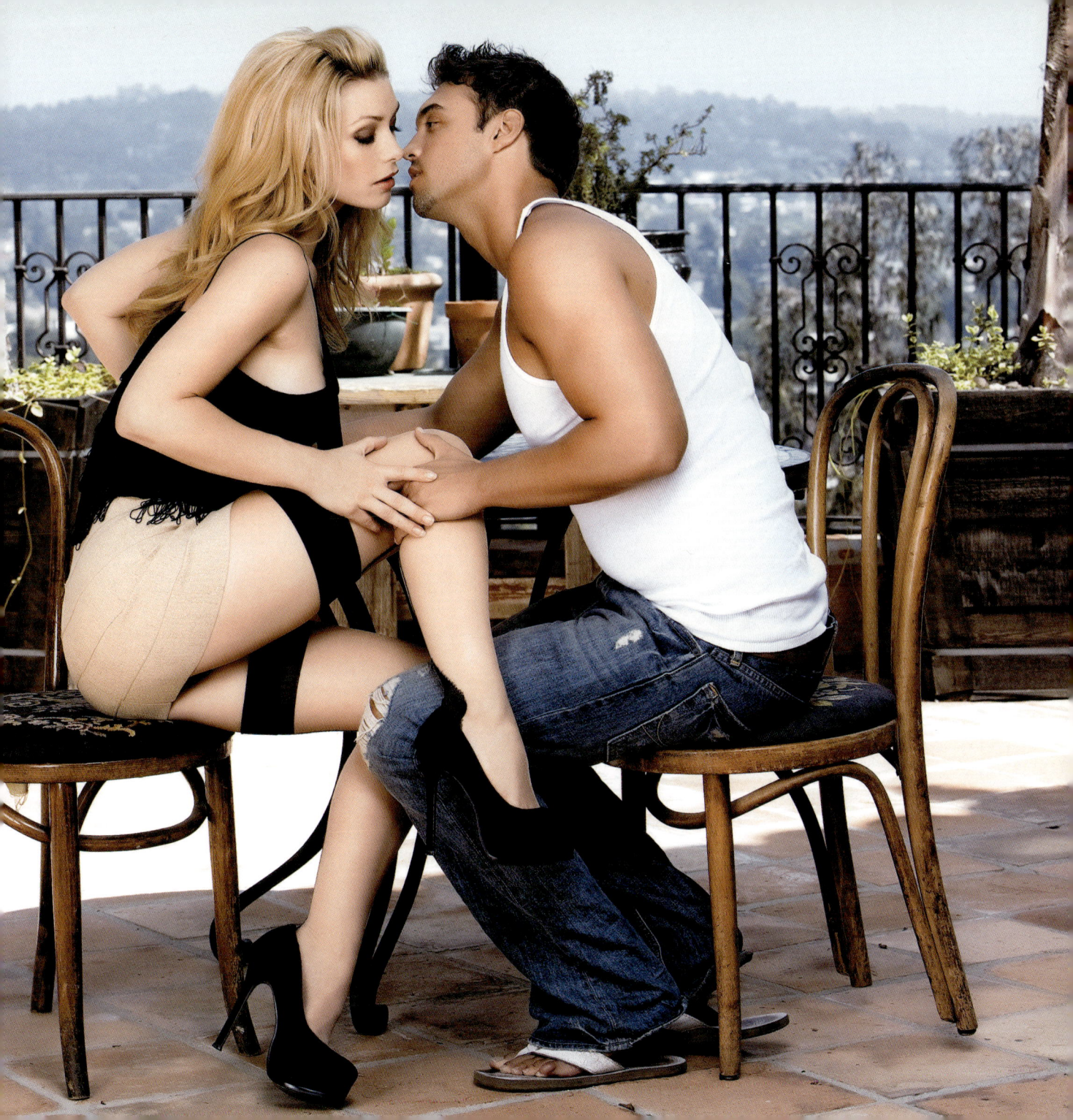

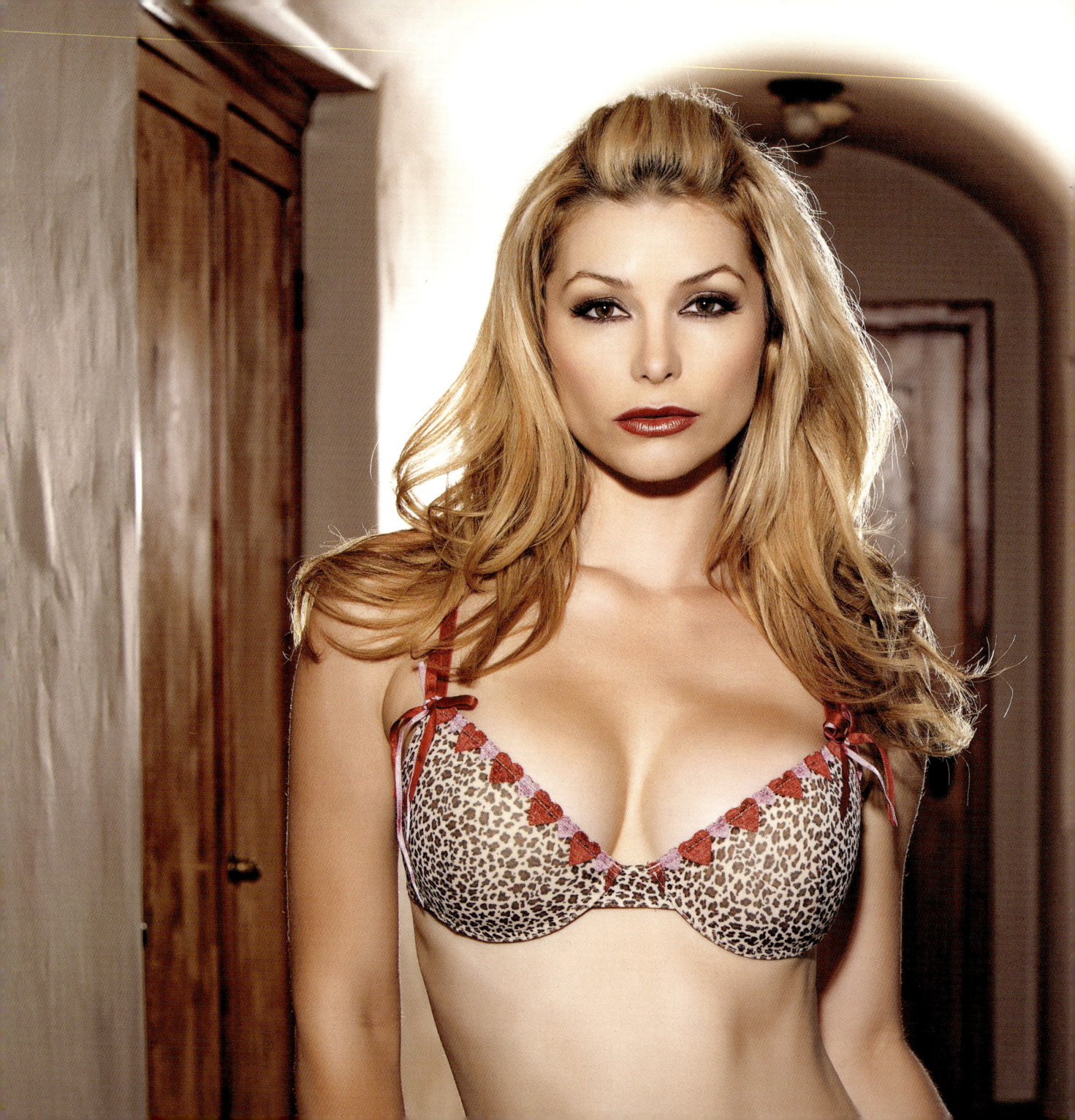

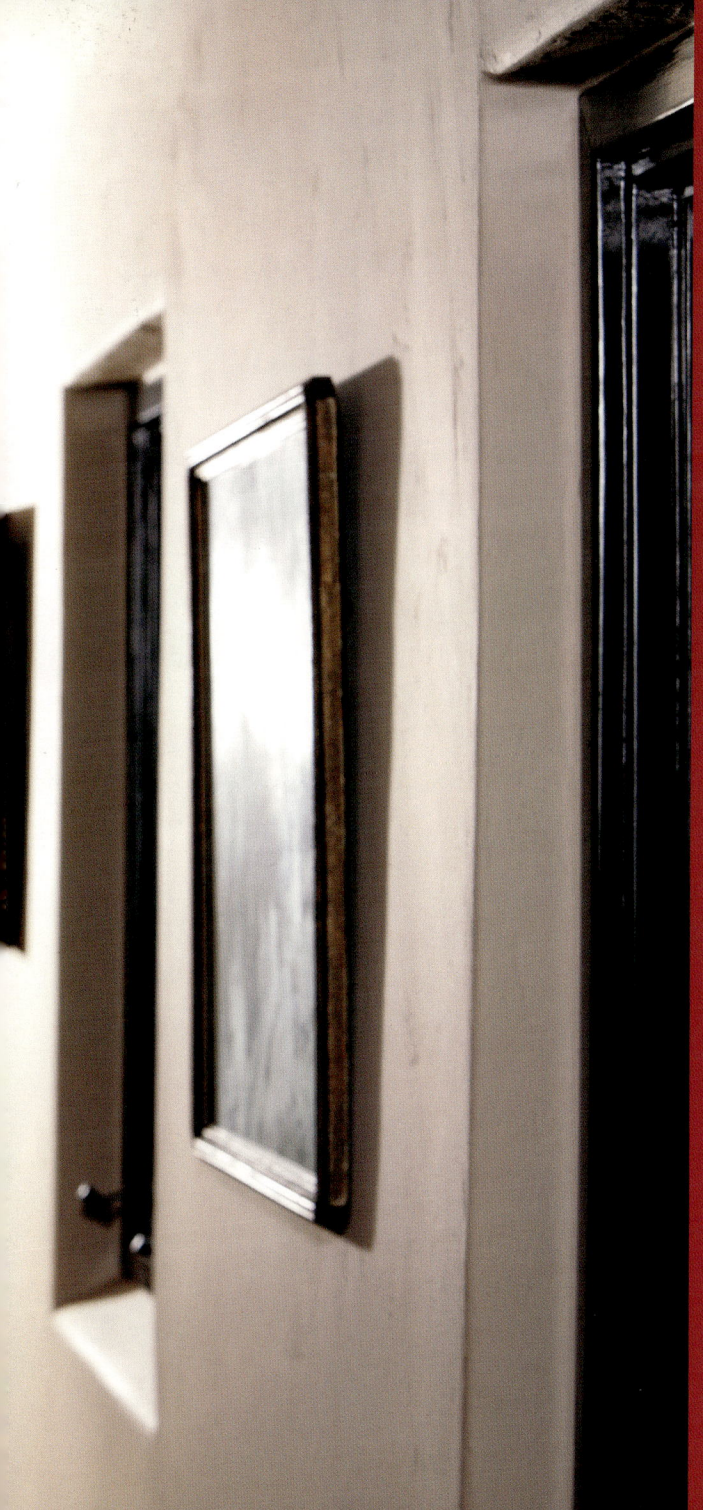

Eye Contact

Before you can make his or her sex throb with desire, you have to break the ice—and eye contact is a great place to start your seduction. Learning to hold someone's gaze—and then how to communicate naughty, sexy thoughts using only your eyes—is the first step. Here are a few specifics to get you started:

Eyes Have It. Try a variety of glances. Start with a bold, unwavering gaze. Then try a wink. And here's a great move: Turn your head away from him but look back out of the corners of your eyes. It's flirtatious and provocative to the max.

Smolder. Have you experienced a "burning" glance? Then you know that the smolder is bolder. Narrow your eyes and focus on a spot just between his. Think hot and naughty thoughts, then purse your lips as if you are a little bit angry. You're sure to get his attention.

Smirk. You're not laughing *at* him . . . just looking a bit amused, even a bit superior. This is the look that says, "I understand you better than anybody in this room—and I can turn *you* on."

Ogle. Start by locking eyes, then look him up and down, lingering over what you like (don't neglect his crotch). Finish with your gaze back at his eyes and hold it there. No disrespect here—just obvious appreciation. Consider this "undressing him with your eyes"—and strip him naked mentally if it helps you telegraph what you're thinking.

Peekaboo. Lower your head so that a lock of your hair falls over one eye (or both eyes), or simply turn your gaze downward. With your head bowed, lift your chin slightly and look up from under your hair. Or try opening your eyes wide and looking up at him—this might be the most flirtatious glance of all.

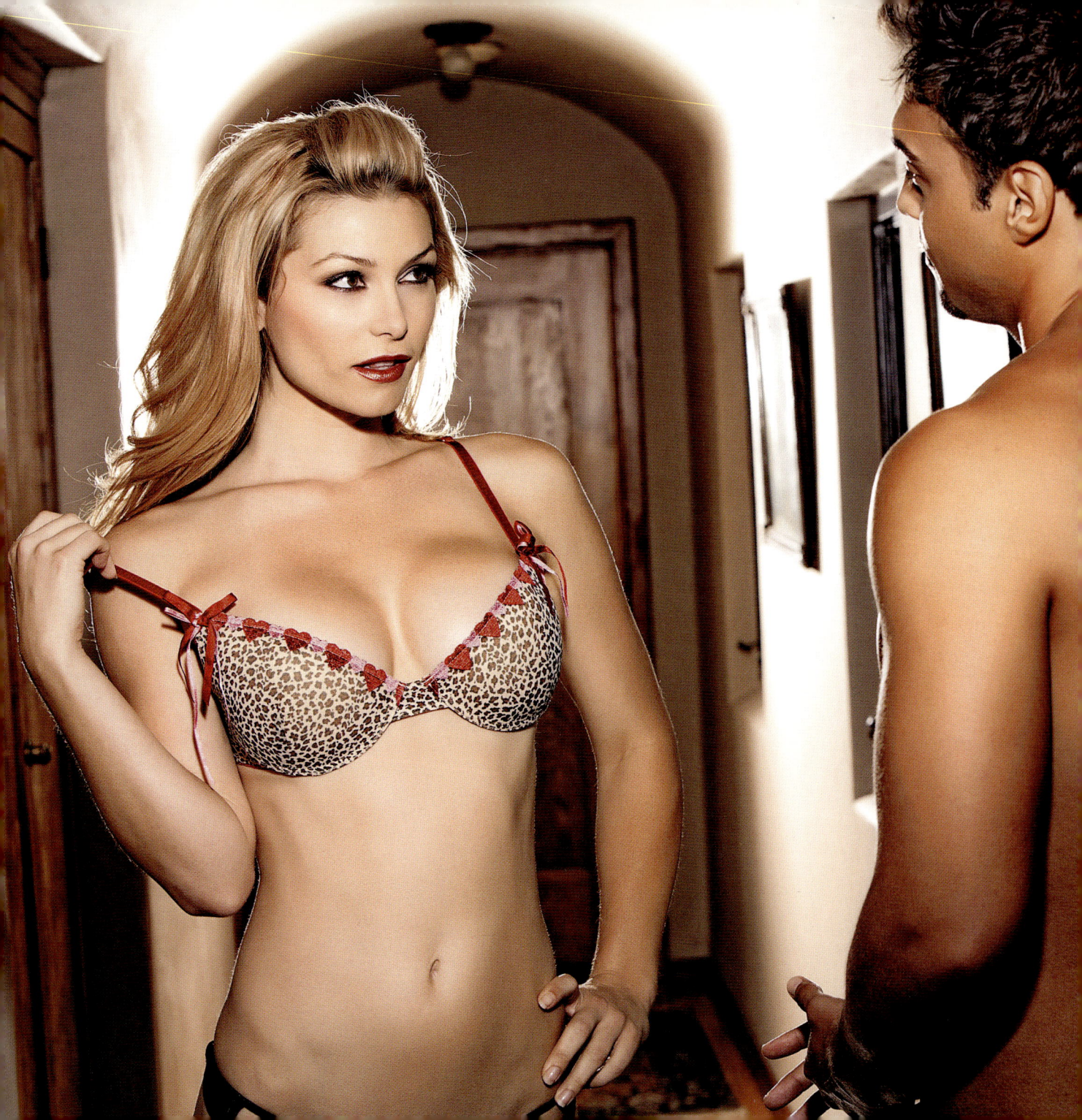

Bodies Talk Louder Than Words

Communicating doesn't just mean speaking in words. Seduction is an all-over affair: Your whole body is talking, so make sure it is saying what you want it to say. Here are some tips for brushing up your body language.

Seduction 101: The Man's Game

Guys, why not try some of these simple ways to make the science of seduction work for you.

Take the "Top" Position. Try to position yourself so that she has to look up at you.

Use Proprietary Touching. As you converse, lightly touch her hand or shoulder, place your palm on her back, or find other ways to touch her that seem as if you are taking charge, taking *care* of her—without being menacing, of course.

Make Eye Contact. It's worth mentioning again: Square off and hold her gaze, exuding a sense of strength and confidence.

Curve Into Her. As things warm up, try to create a "crook" with your body so that your arm is behind hers and her shoulder rests near your armpit. This is another protective gesture she'll respond to without even thinking about it.

Cock Your Head. A scrutinizing type of expression can be very sexy. She'll feel exposed—and that's a good thing, assuming all is moving along nicely.

Put Ankle to Knee. When you sit, cross your legs so that one ankle is resting on the other knee. This subtle, crotch-exposing gesture shows a sexy openness.

Rest Hands on Waist. Stand with your hands on the back of your waist, gently pushing your hips forward. This is another "come hither" gesture. (But make sure your pants aren't *too* tight, unless you want to come off like a Chippendale's guy.)

Seduction 101: The Woman's Game

Just like the guys, there are things you can do to make chemistry work for you, even if flirting doesn't come as naturally as walking and talking. Here are a few surefire ways to get under his skin—without his realizing you are doing a thing:

Face Up to It. All of the flirting techniques listed here constitute a kind of body language—so make those glances, gazes, and winks part of your overall body movement. He'll focus on your face above all, so be sure you are superanimated.

Smile. It sounds obvious, but if you want to light up the room, don't forget to turn on your brights. Try different smiles, too: smirky, appreciative, skeptical—whatever makes you feel and seem lively and engaged.

Open for Business. Keep your body language wide open—but not your legs. A sexy cross at the knees will show off your calves and ankles. Avoid crossing your arms across your chest; instead, use them to gesture during your conversation. Lean forward slightly from the waist, whether you are sitting or standing, as if drawn to him.

Use Your Hands. While men should touch their dates in small ways, you should touch *yourself*. Stroke your own neck, cup your face in your hand, play with your jewelry, smooth your stocking, play with the zipper of your boot . . . all of this will make him wish he were a glove on your hand. Be careful not to fidget, though—keep your movements sly, deliberate, and seductive.

Involve Your Body. Circle your foot, run a finger around the rim of your glass, lick your lips, toss or twirl your hair, play with your buttons . . . Don't overdo this stuff, but a bit of movement will keep him riveted to you and wondering what *else* you can do.

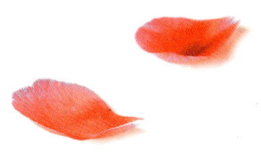

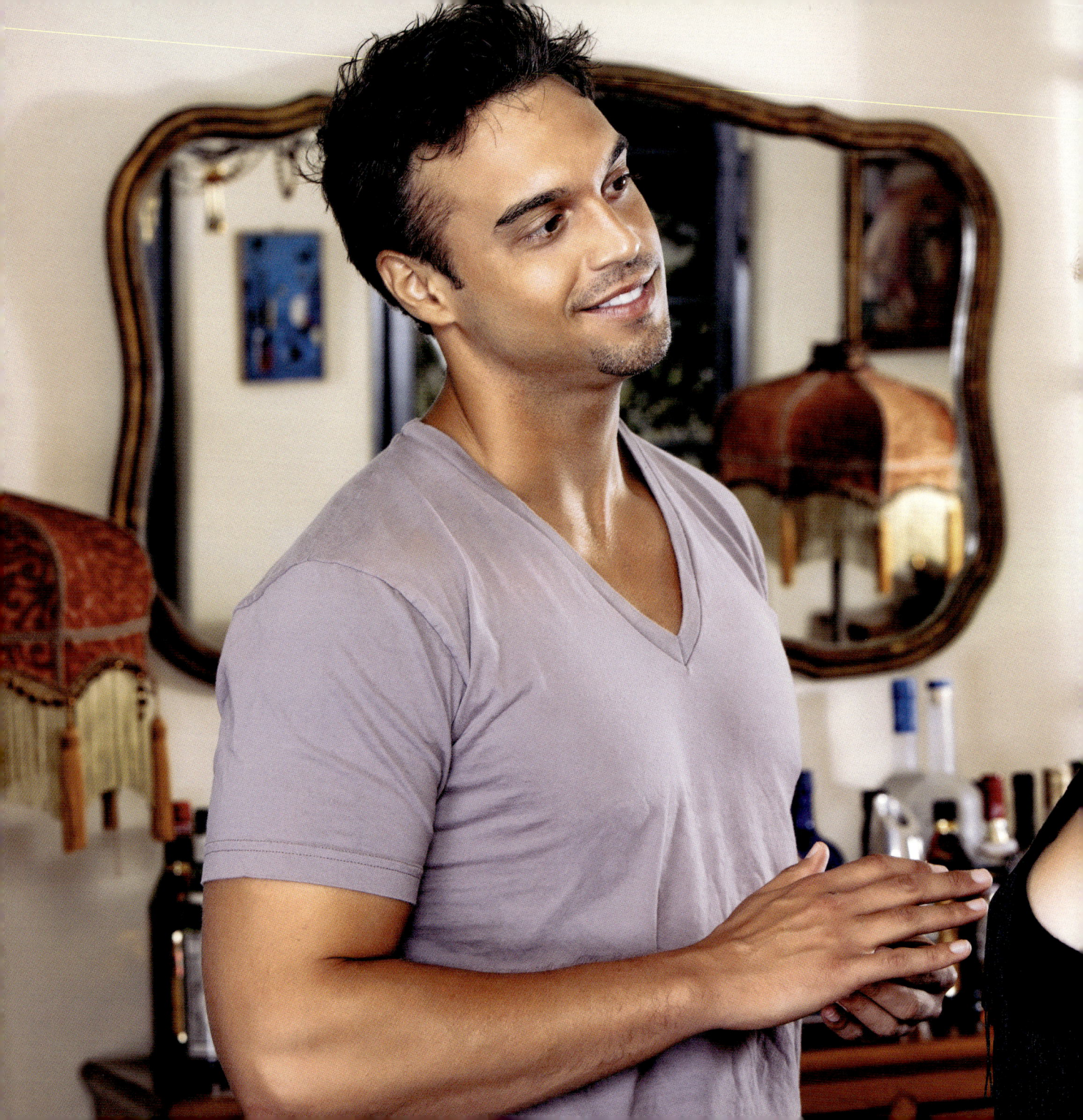

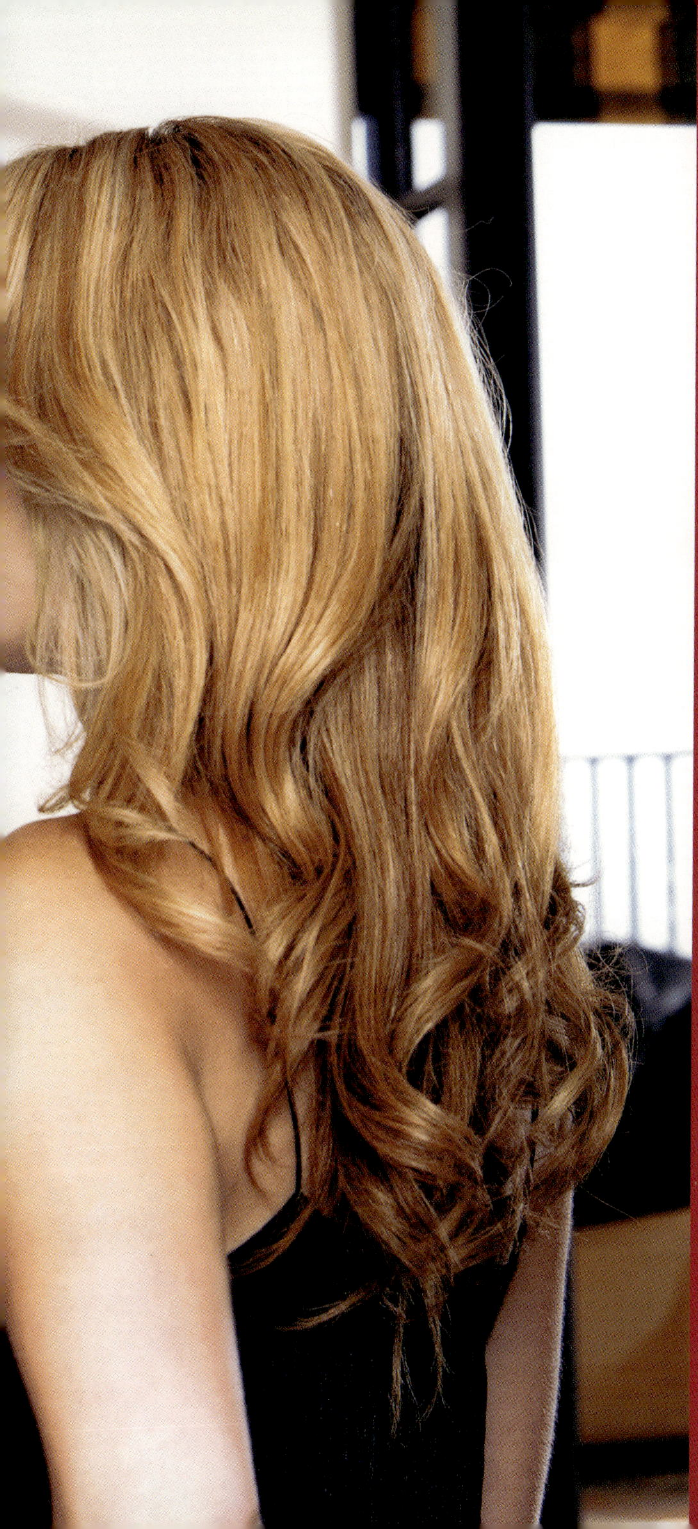

Other Moves. Don't be afraid to involve every inch of yourself in the seduction: Stretch, arch your back, and feel free to invade his space so that you can bring your speaking volume down to a whisper. No matter how civilized the setting, some unexpectedly bold moves on your part can surprise and please the object of your attention. It's all in good, sexy fun.

Use Your Words. Suggestive comments can seal the deal—especially in a public setting, where you have to keep your voices low and exhibit self-control to keep your hands off each other. Whispers, murmurs . . . if you want to play the sex kitten, don't forget to purr.

Sparkle. Keep the content of your small talk light, fun, and agreeable. Use innuendo and double entendres. Clever humor can be very sexy. Ask questions and really listen to his answers. Since all of flirtation and foreplay is about responsiveness, be responsive—but don't be afraid to disagree. There's nothing wrong with a bit of feisty independence (even playing hard to get) along with your femininity, as long as you don't come off as cranky or dismissive.

Move in and Touch. Stand close to him and touch his shoulder, chest, arm, back, or even thigh. Keep your touch light and feathery—promising and gentle—or run a fingernail up his arm or back to suggest a stronger touch. Stroke his thigh, finger his belt, even run your hands down his back and cup his ass. Or, if it suits you better, be more understated in your touch: Hold his hand, stroke his wrist, and use innocent touches to build anticipation for what is to come.

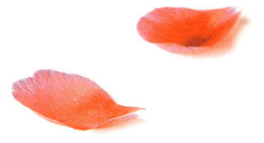

Put On—or Turn Off—the Pressure. Think of your seduction style as having three flavors: aggressive, submissive, and hard to get. You may have a favorite, but try each one in turn or mix the three—and always try to read your partner to see which he responds to most readily.

Feeling aggressive? Try backing him into a corner, using a firm touch, and flirting more suggestively. Some men love a sense of being forcibly "taken," and if he's one of them, a little assertiveness might be just the thing to set the night on fire.

If you are in a submissive mood, use those shy flirting techniques: Keep your hands behind your back, tilt your head, speak quietly, ask lots of questions, and agree with him readily. He'll get the message that he's in charge, and he'll relish the opportunity.

Some guys thrive on pursuit. If that's your guy, back off and let him take the lead. Lean away and let him move in. Back up and let him move forward. Check out other guys in the room. Sometimes, the best "come hither" move is a bit of distance and a dose of cool.

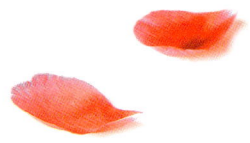

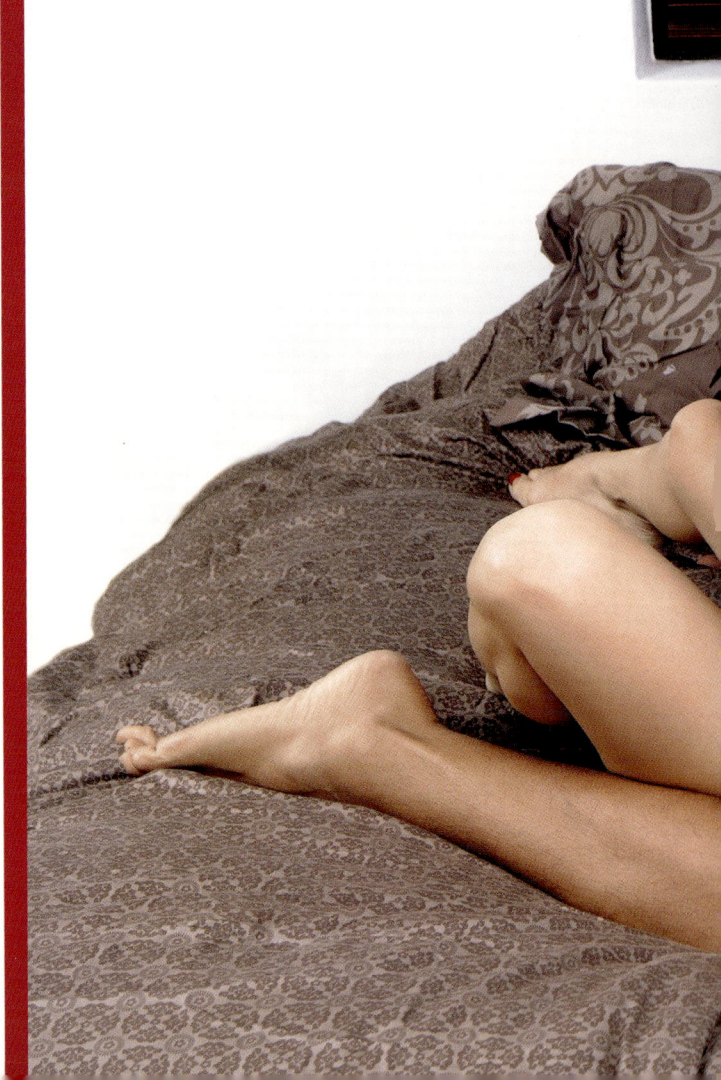

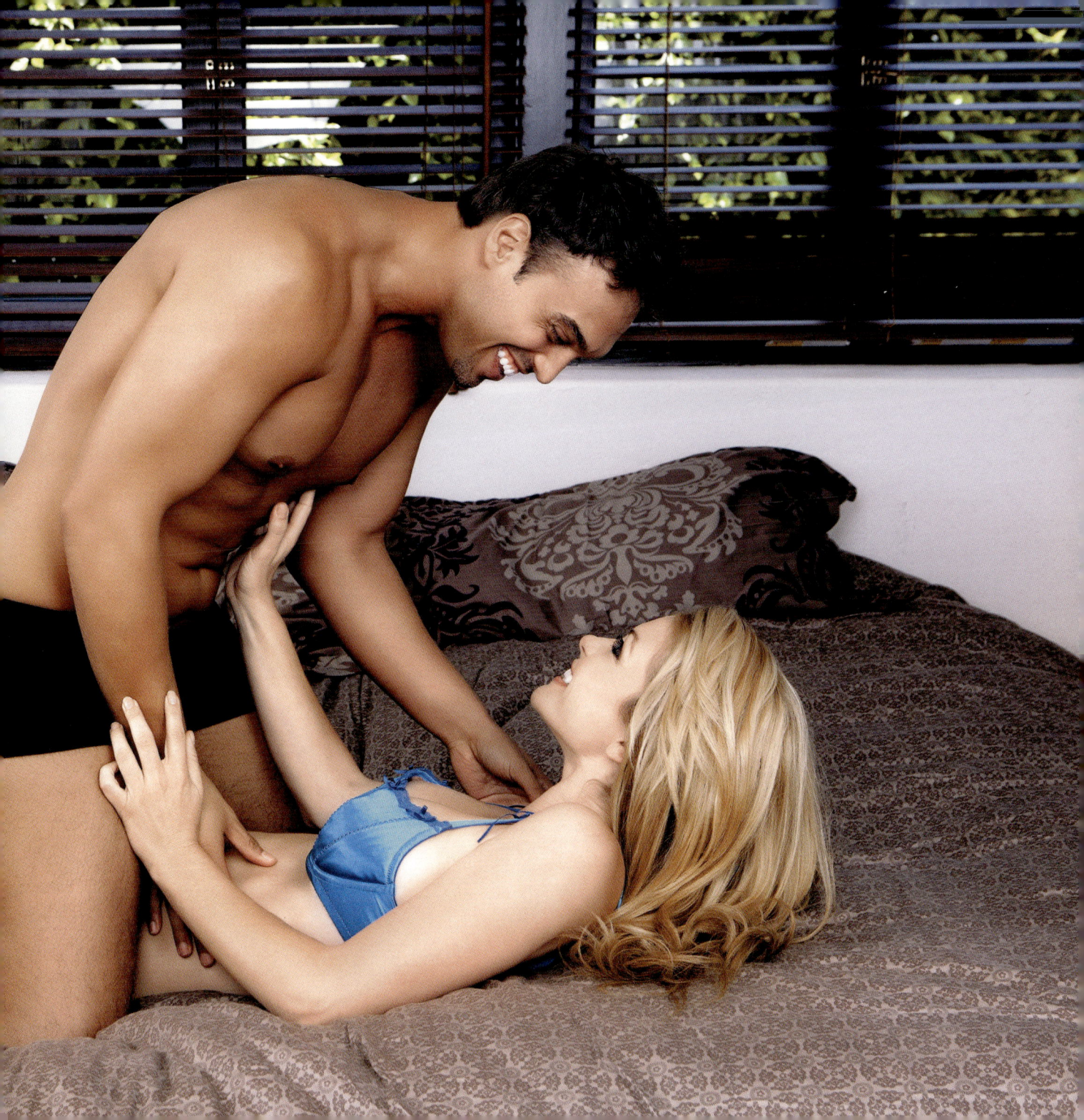

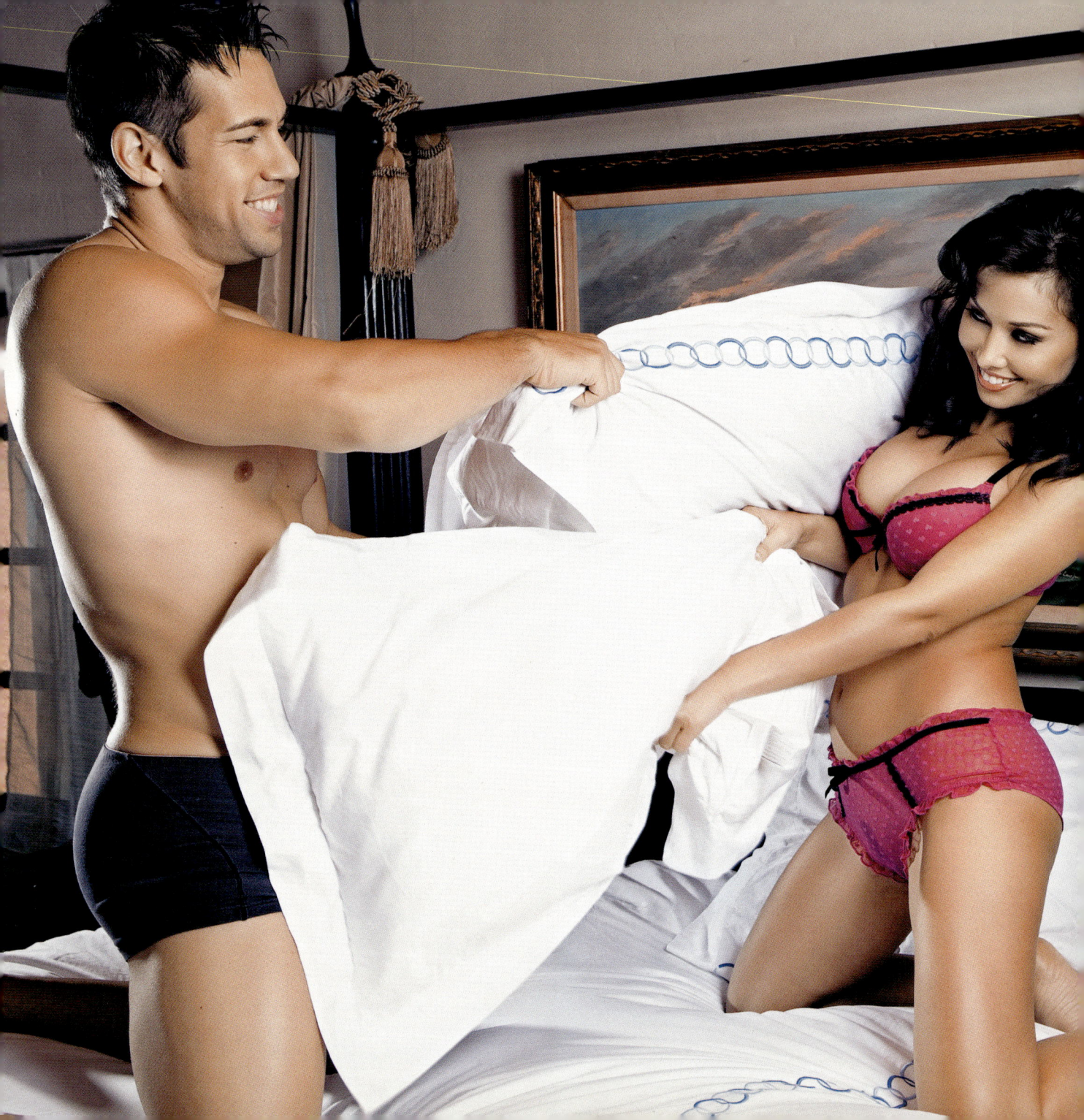

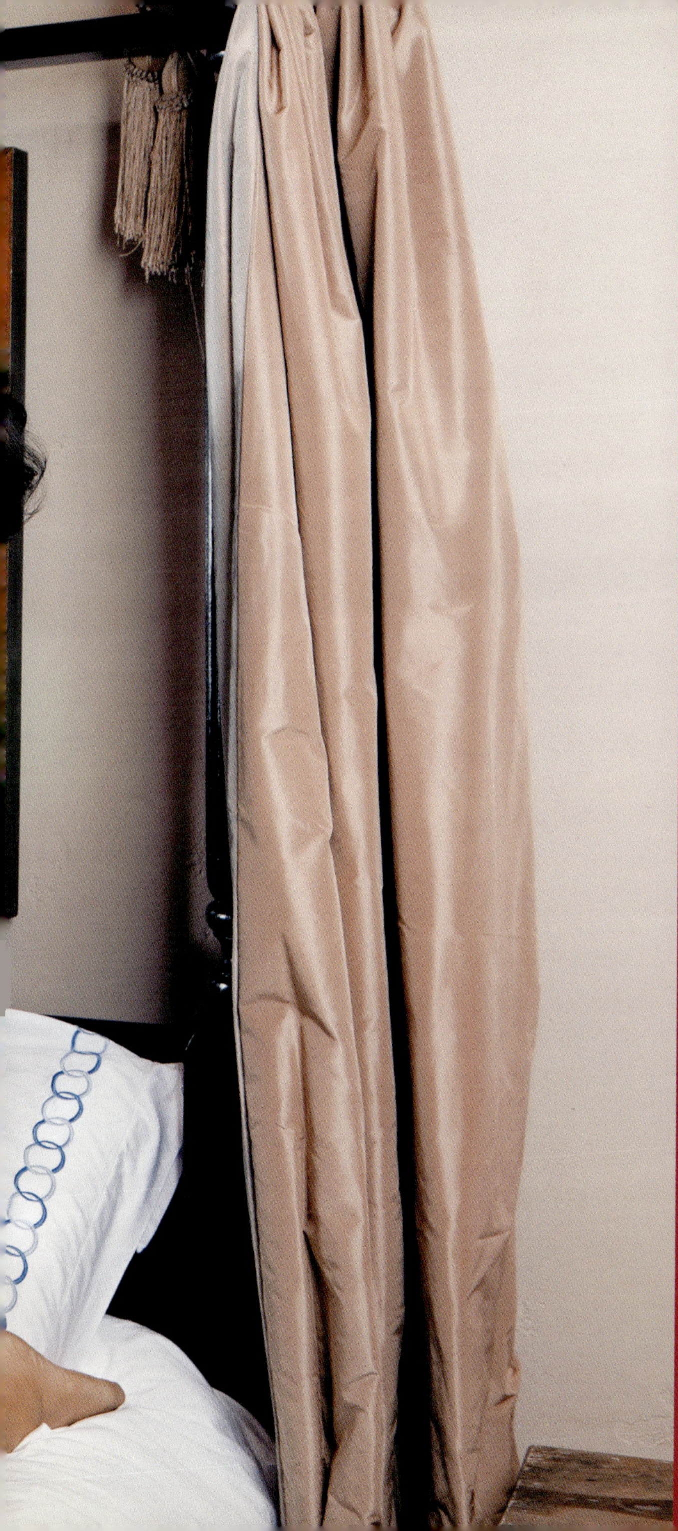

Getting Your Hearts Racing

Heart-racing, blood-pumping fun—that's what great sex is all about. And getting that heart going is part of foreplay. Here are a few activities that can add to the mood:

Chase each other around the room, around the house, even around the block. Once you catch her, wrap your arms around her and kiss her boldly. This suggestive hint of capture and restraint may work like a match on a pile of tinder.

Tickle each other—not to the point of pain, but just so you are both having fun. Shared laughter is essential for feeling close—not to mention, tickling gets your hands on his body.

Have a race. Biking, running, swimming . . . a bit of friendly competition can make you hot for each other: The winner gets to rip the loser's clothes off.

Have a pillow fight. Connecting with your inner child just might bring out the X-rated grownup in you.

Scare each other—playfully, of course. Jump out from behind the couch, sneak up behind your lover and whisper "Boo," toss a pillow and yell "Heads up!" Assuming you both have strong hearts, a little startling fun never hurts.

Have a wrestling match. Chances are your man is stronger than you—but there's something very sexy about trying to pin him, escape his grasp, or wriggle out from under him.

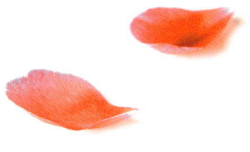

Calm Down

On the other side of the coin, sometimes life is just too hectic or too stressful to feel sexy. At those times, it's best to come up with ways to calm down together, slow the pace, focus on each other, and fan the flames of passion slowly:

Kill the lights. Everything is sexier by candlelight, so dim it down, slow it down, and enjoy the mood. Showering together with the lights off can be both relaxing and supremely sexy—give it a try.

Cue the music. Skip the hard rock and select some new age, folk, or classical music to unwind by. Nothing sets the tone like just the right mix of tunes played at a volume that allows for quiet conversation.

Contact. Gentle play, light stroking, or delicious mutual massage (start with those tired feet or that aching head) will get your bodies humming in tune. Tamp down the sexual energy for now and concentrate on relaxing and renewing each other with loving caresses.

Relax your posture. Have him lay his head in your lap and let him doze off for a minute or two while you stroke his hair. Or curl up together and take a cat nap—then take advantage of that sleepy, drowsy feeling when you wake up to snuggle closer and nuzzle his neck.

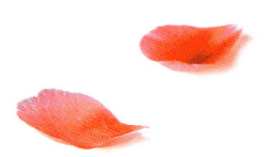

Start the Day with Zing

If you want to drive your lover crazy all day long, ring his chimes as he's leaving the house in the morning. Don't just kiss him good-bye—give him a supersexy, sweet-tasting, tongue-twisting smackeroo that says you'll be eagerly awaiting his return. He'll be distracted all day long—and by the time he comes home, he just might be able to ring the doorbell with his hands full. Alternatively, use one of the techniques outlined in chapter 2, 3, or 4—such as fondling his ass, waking him up by sucking on his penis, leaving a trail of kisses from his neck to the top of his crack, or just flashing your bare breasts—to remind him of things to come.

Here are a few other ways to keep the flirtation going when you aren't there:

Slip a sexy note into his briefcase, telling him in detail exactly what you want to do to him when he gets home from work. Add a postscript telling him that the thought of stroking his stiff cock will keep you turned on all day, too.

Shoot a revealing snapshot of yourself in a seductive or naughty pose—and stick it in his suit jacket pocket before he leaves the house. Try fondling your breasts or putting your hand in your panties in the shot. He'll get the picture.

Leave him a hot phone message on his private work line that will be waiting for him when he gets in (or when he returns from lunch)—or on his cell phone, if privacy is a concern. Mention one of your favorite techniques—such as running your tongue around the tip of his cock or tugging on his testicles—so there's no doubt about what's to come.

Send him sexy texts. Why should teenagers have a monopoly on "sexting"? Let a grown-up show how it's done, and get your lover's blood rushing to his thumbs as he matches you innuendo for innuendo. Or address your text message to his cock—and tell it just how much you adore teasing it with your tongue.

Take It Off—in Style

Before we leave the subject of seduction, let's take it all off. That's right, I'm talking about the art of the striptease. What could be more of a come-on than a personal show performed for your lover's pleasure? Especially when it is followed by a down-to-business lap dance.

To pull off a great striptease (and gentlemen, you are by no means exempt from this form of fun), you have to call upon those reserves of self-confidence. If it helps, pretend you are playing a role—you aren't *yourself*, you're Lola (or Lawrence) the stripper. Sip on a glass of wine to relax, then use whatever mind game gets you in the mood to reveal yourself in a slow, scintillating dance of seduction.

Select your music for maximum effect, something you can move to that you will both enjoy. The important part is that you've thought about it and set it up so you can make a grand entrance.

Practice by yourself, in front of a mirror, so you can work out your best moves. Put the music on and let your body flow with it in whatever way feels natural to you. (Later, if you want, you can strip in front of the mirror so you can both watch.)

Set up a viewing area, then decide if you want him dressed or completely naked, tied to the chair or free to use his hands. If you're turned on by his reaction, consider making him strip first so you can watch his cock harden and throb as you perform your moves.

Dress for a successful undress. In other words, layer on the garments, keeping in mind how they'll look coming off. Gloves, scarves, and high-heeled pumps are great accessories for the ladies and will help you prolong the tease a little bit. Be creative as you explore your closet—wear a long black jacket over a sexy bra, leave off the underwear but slip on killer heels, or pull your top down to reveal your breasts, then tie a sheer scarf over

them for a sensual see-through effect. Gentlemen, think about shirts you can pull open easily (over the head isn't very sexy) and pants that'll drop to the floor on cue. And every seducer and seductress should have top-notch undergarments in sexy colors such as red and black—and show them off whenever he or she gets the chance.

Take it easy and use your hands. Keep your moves slow and sensual and use your hands throughout, running them over your crotch or belly, enjoying the way you feel, calling attention to your best assets. Touch your breasts or chest and your waist, embrace yourself, lean over and show off your ass. Exaggerate your movements—undulate, twist, and sway to the music.

Use your hair. This one is more for the ladies: Don't forget to toss your hair, caress it, whip it around—even whip your lover with it. Bend over and let your hair sweep the floor, then flip it back to show your beautiful face.

Get hip. Your hips are the centerpiece of your sensuality, so use them to the max in your striptease. Roll them, shake them back and forth, thrust them, and show them off from every angle. A preview of what you can do with that pelvis will have your lover panting for more.

Use your squatter's rights. Rather than remaining on your feet, try squatting as you thrust out your behind, or use a chair as a prop: Straddle it, sit sideways, throw your legs over the back, and use it as a "partner" in your dance.

Put on a peep show. Here's a fun twist: Instead of performing your show right out in the open for him, find a door with an open keyhole. Make him kneel in front of the keyhole and watch you through it. (If your house has only solid doors, position him outside of a first-floor window—but be aware that you might be putting on a show for the neighbors, as well!) Pretend you think you're alone, getting undressed without knowing anyone is watching. If there is a Peeping Tom in him, this will drive him wild.

Follow up by getting physical. Once the clothes are off, try a sensual lap dance. Straddle your lover and put on your best moves. Soon everyone's clothes will be on the floor (or possibly the chandelier).

Take a field trip. If you are apprehensive about the whole stripping thing (or if you find yourselves obsessed with it), go to a strip club or a Chippendales show (if you want something a bit campier and more comical) together sometime. Watching the pros might loosen you up and provide some handy ideas—and the steamy atmosphere is sure to turn you both on. Gentlemen, watch the dancers to your heart's content but remember that your own beautiful lady is by your side, so be sure to involve her in your fantasies. Stroke and caress her as you watch the action, and whisper in her ear which moves you'd like to see *her* perform. Ladies, enjoy the show and take mental notes. Let your man know that you find the whole thing as sexy as he does. And if you two are really feeling adventurous (and have a few extra dollars), pay for a private "couple's dance" and get some personal attention.

Still think that foreplay begins in the bedroom? There's so much sexy fun to be had when you let your inner flirt emerge and take over the preliminaries. Seduction is half the fun, after all, and it can make the bedroom part of the evening that much hotter when you finally get there.

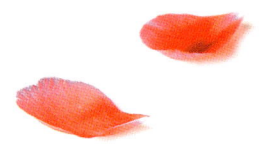

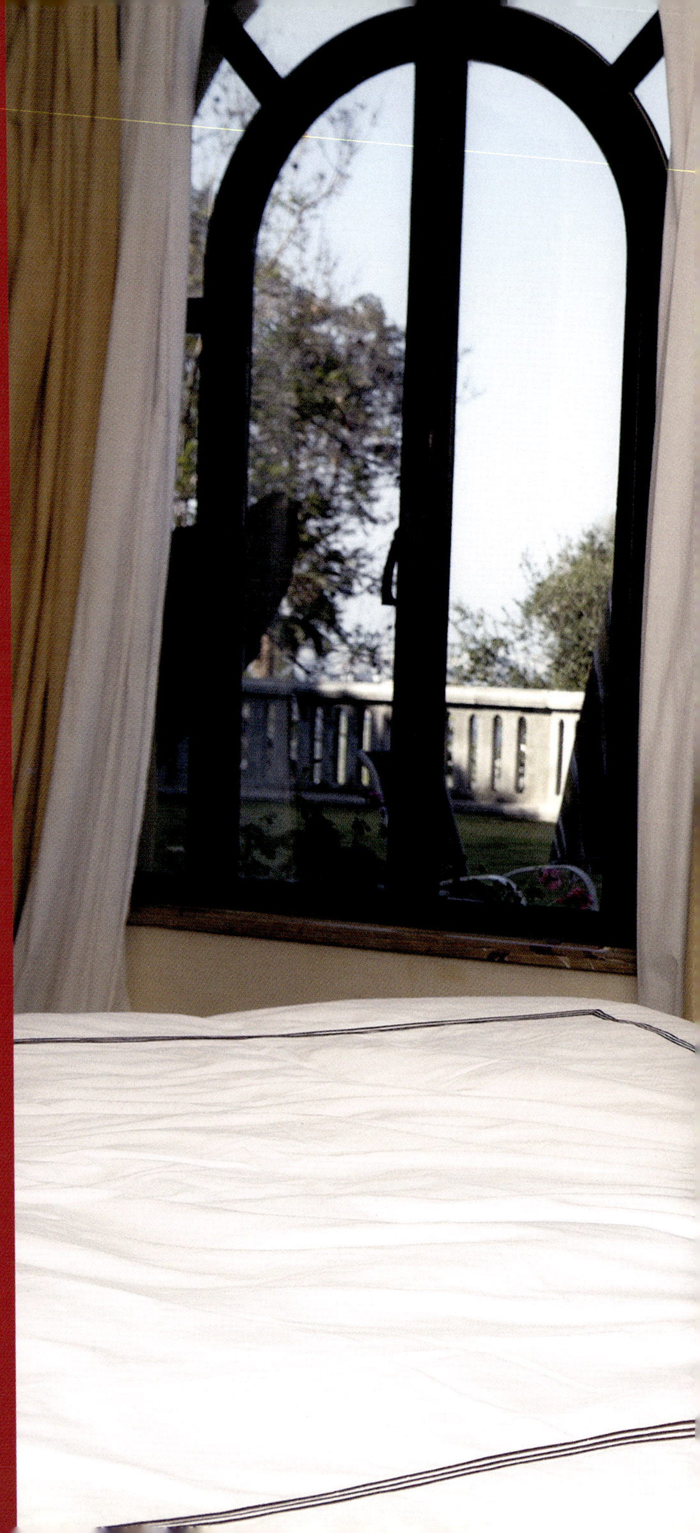

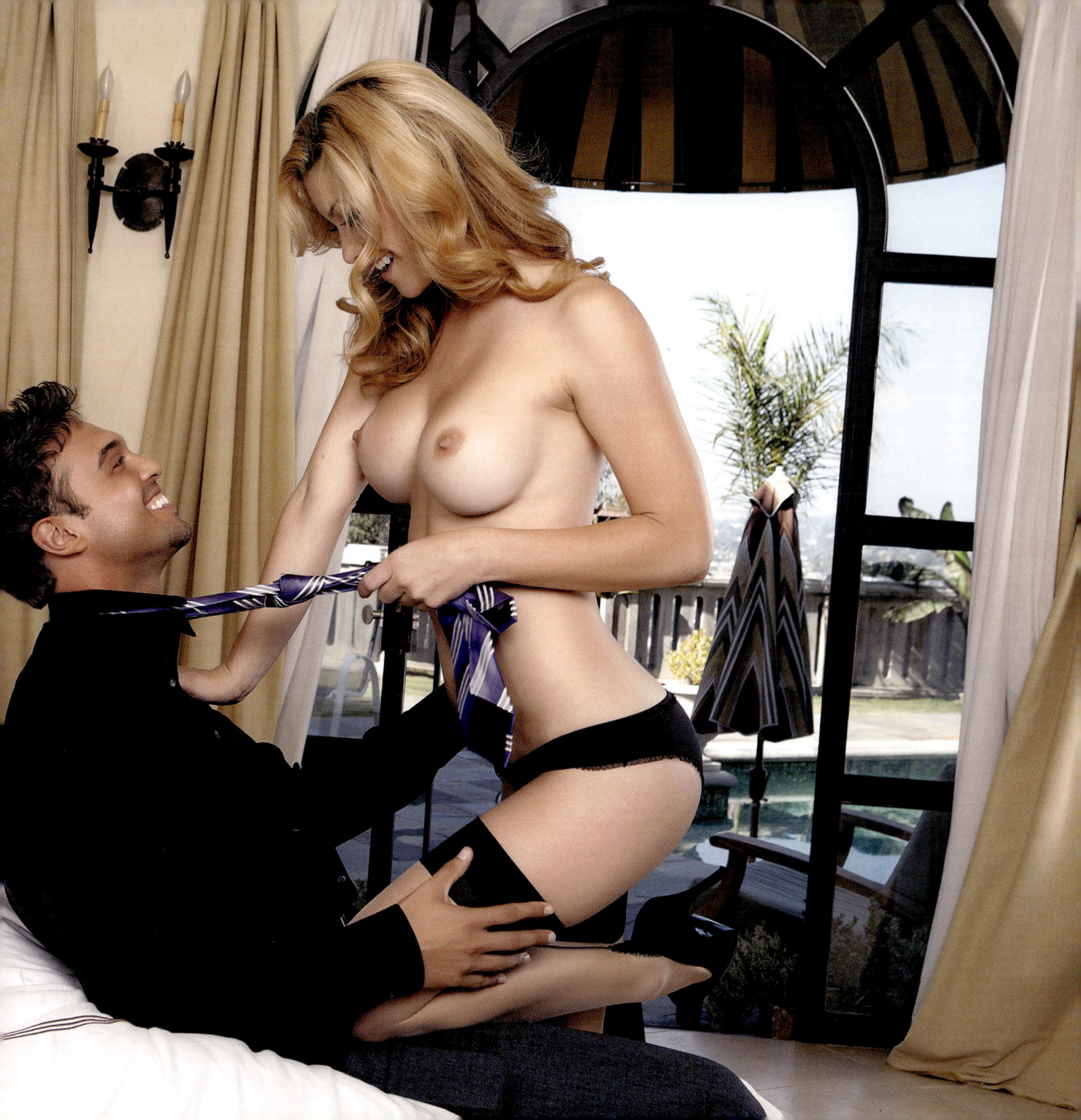

Creative Kissing and More with Mouths

Is there anything in the world more thrilling than locking lips with your lover in a deep, deliciously passionate soul kiss? For most of us, kissing is the launchpad to intimacy—the moment when communication becomes literally oral, when our conversation transcends words and our bodies start to think and speak for themselves. Kissing is the natural starting point for foreplay, and there's a lot to be said for making an art of it.

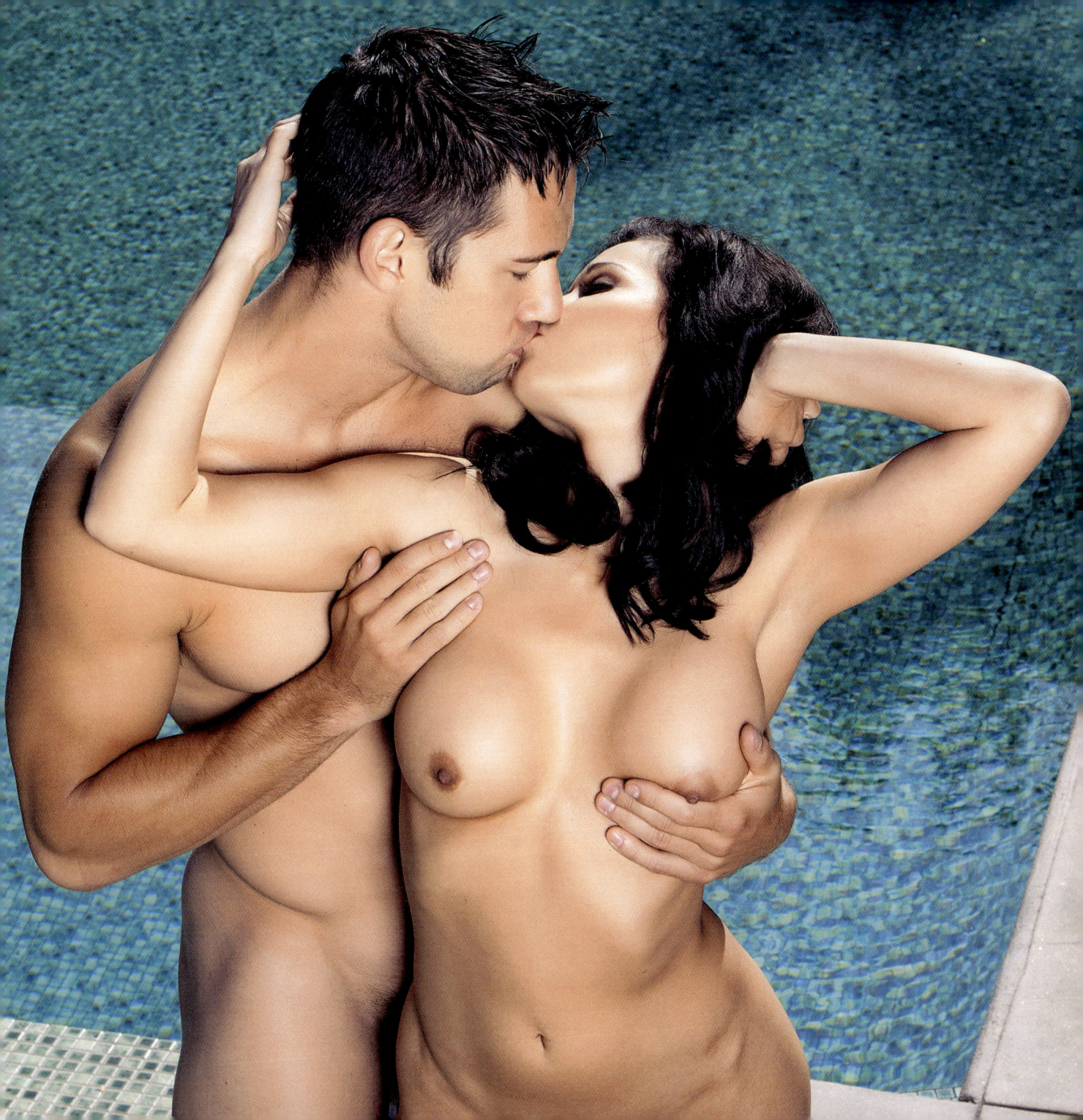

Sealed with a Kiss

Some people enjoy hours and hours of kissing—remember when we called it "making out"?—and see this soulful pastime as an end in itself. But for most of us, it is part of the warm-up for sex (and part of the main event, too, of course). How many different kinds of mouth-to-mouth kisses can you think of, off the top of your head? Perhaps we've come up with a few you haven't focused on. Try them all, see what you both enjoy, and remember to change it up often! You'll hear this a few more times throughout the book—and it bears repeating: Variety makes foreplay more interesting, more surprising, and more fun. (And it should go without saying, but we'll say it: Never neglect your oral hygiene, and be absolutely sure your breath is kissing sweet.)

Let's start with our own favorite mouth-to-mouth kisses:

The Featherlight. Relax your mouth and part your lips just slightly. Using just the tips of your lips, brush over your lover's lips and then pull away. Go in again for a few more gentle brushes, then try a small nibble by grabbing first his upper lip, then his lower one, with the very tips of your own lips—then letting go. (Think of this as a fish nibble.) Use the very tip of your tongue to gently press into the corner of his mouth, just to tease him a little bit about the deeper kisses to come.

Firm but Friendly. When movie stars embrace for that final, burning on-screen kiss, they make it look as if they are exploring one another's mouths with their tongues—but in fact it wouldn't look very appetizing if they were. Instead, they go for a firm, intimate—but dry—smooch. This kind of kiss can be very sexy and, again, a great promise of what's to come. Move in on your partner and encircle her upper body in a close embrace. Tilt your head slightly, relax and part your lips just a little bit, and plant a firm, lingering kiss on her mouth—the kind that shows you are in charge. If she starts to move in with her tongue, cup her face with your hands and pull away for a few seconds to let her know you want to take it slow and steady. (This refrain will become familiar throughout the course of this book: Holding back, rather than rushing ahead, can be *great* foreplay.)

The Explorer. Yes, it is time for your tongues to meet—but again, take a small step and leave yourself some room to escalate. Allow your lips to meet in a relaxed kiss and then gently open your mouth wider to allow your tongue to explore his. Don't jam your tongue into his mouth, though; just go in part way, allowing your tongue to search for his and probe it a little bit. Circle the tip of his tongue with yours, explore his teeth lightly, check under his tongue with the tip of yours—then pull back out again, as you let him reciprocate.

Journey to the Center of the Earth. You are undoubtedly starting to feel the warm glow that delicious kisses inspire, and now you want to explore your lover's mouth to the fullest. Go right ahead, but with some finesse. (When asked to describe their experiences of bad kissing, women invariably cite the "tongue jammers" who nearly choke them with overenthusiastic thrusting and twisting.) Think of your tongue as a lithe seal swimming gracefully into her mouth, exploring the nooks and crannies with the tip, the sides, even the underside. Meet her tongue and get to know it, teasingly, creatively. The soulful, classic French kiss, executed well, is a delightfully mutual exchange of sensations, a kind of dance inside your mouths—and don't forget to vary your lip pressure continually, first pressing harder, then letting up slightly and repositioning your mouth. Constant movement is the hallmark of great soul kissing (and great foreplay in general). You could spend hours enjoying this one.

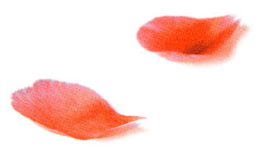

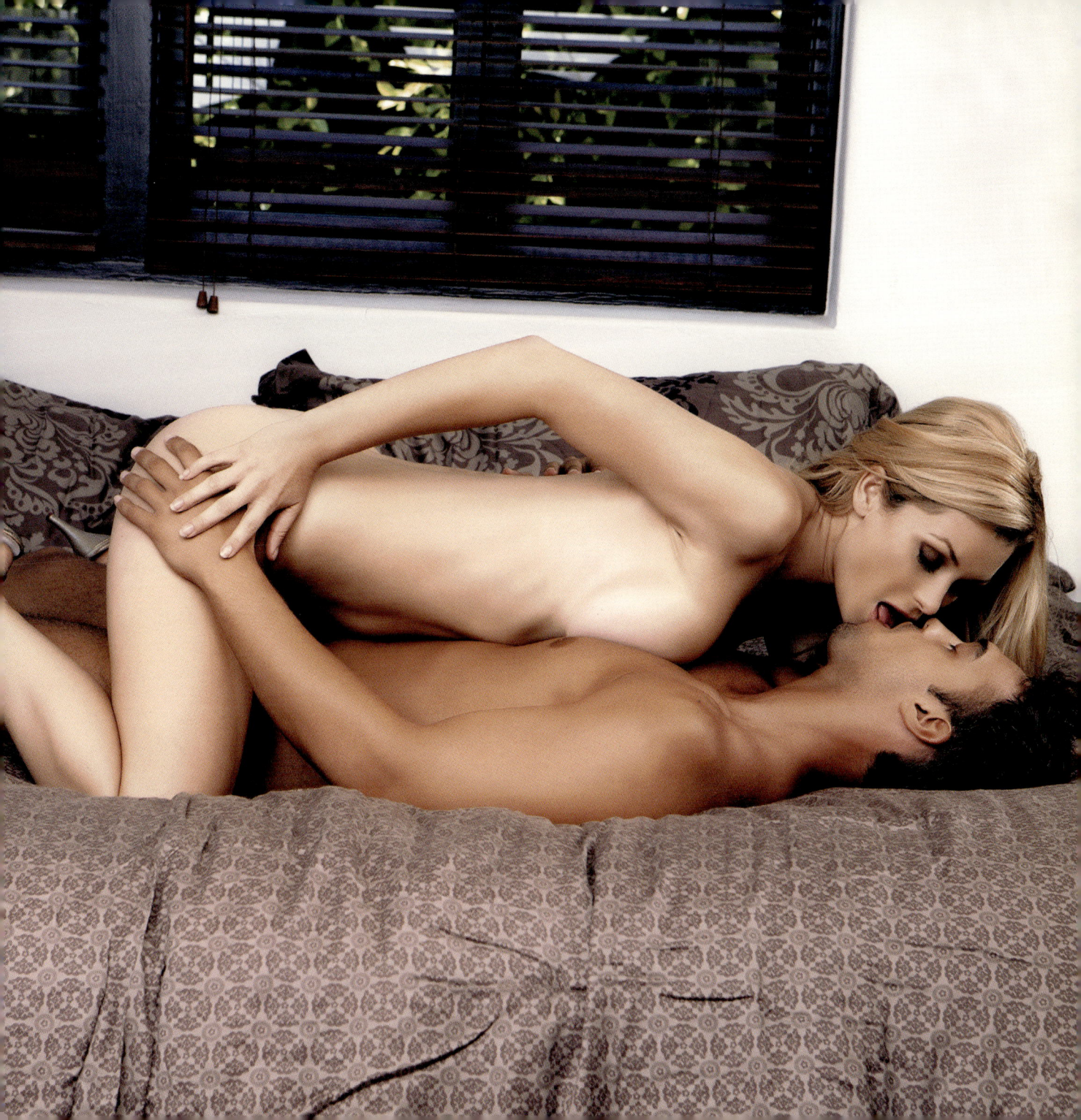

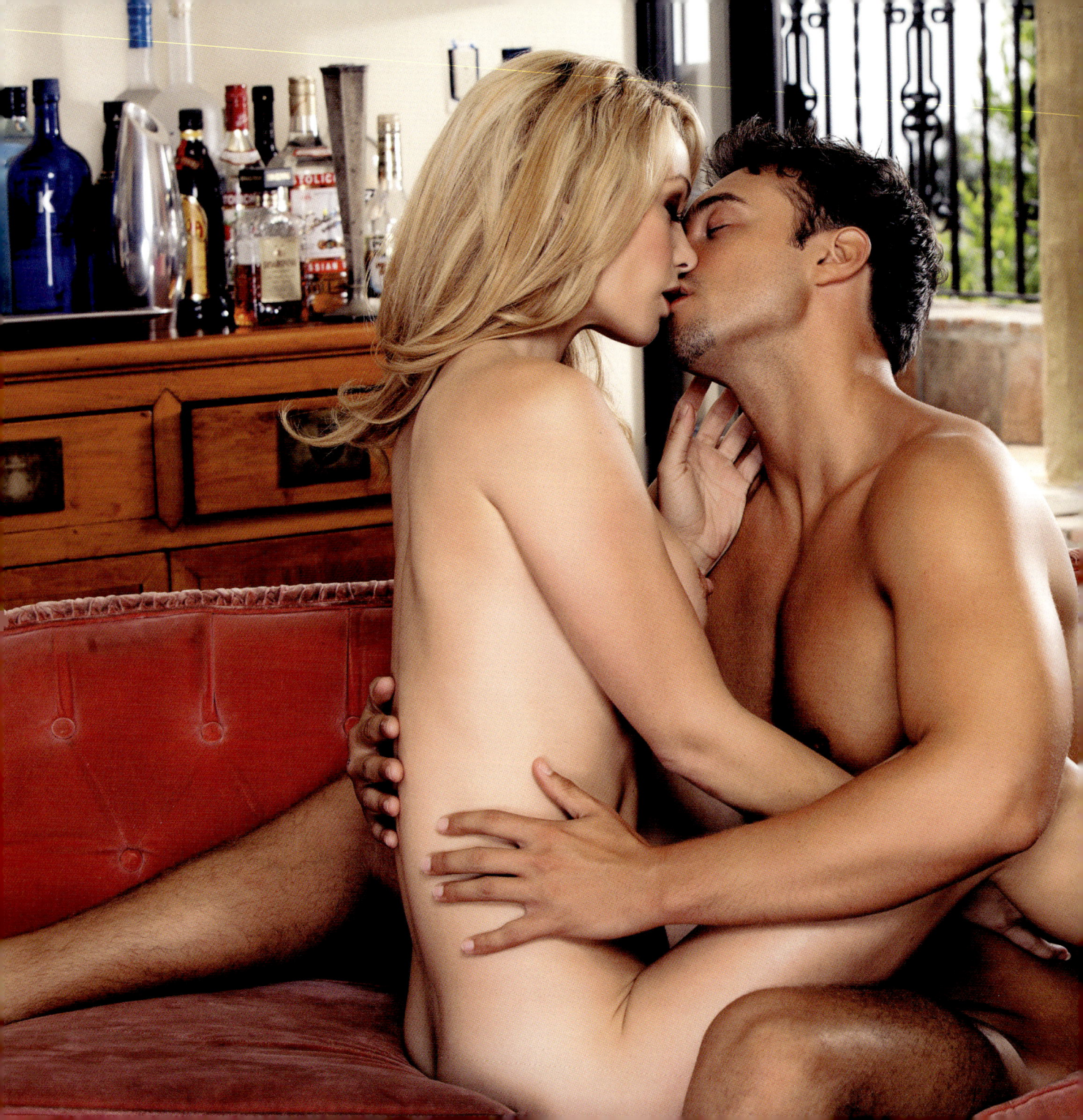

The Hoover. This kiss is a matter of taste: Some find it a bit intense, but it can be highly erotic, so we suggest using it as a variation on the more straightforward techniques. Position your lips around his so that his lips are just slightly inside yours. Press against him firmly and exert gentle suction so his lips are pulled gently into your mouth. After a few seconds, release him and gently flick the tip of your tongue in a circle around his lips. These sensations in alternation will make his heart flutter and bring him in for more. (There's no real blowing in a blow job— or in kissing, either. But sucking is another matter entirely!) Alternatively, take one of his lips into your mouth and suck it ever so gently; move to another part of the lip and repeat.

Swirl and Switch. When it comes to kissing, doing what comes naturally will take you pretty far—but learning a few tricks can be fun, too. This one, first described in ancient Eastern erotica, will wake up your partner's mouth for sure (and it'll work like a charm on her nether regions, as well, when the time comes). During a French kiss (the basis for the Explorer and Journey to the Center of the Earth, described earlier in this section), start swirling your tongue around her mouth, from the roof to the sides, to under the tongue, as if you are gently washing it. After several revolutions, alternate with a decisive poking motion into her mouth (not too deeply.), then return to the swirl. Watch her reaction to discover whether she is enjoying it and just the right amount of pressure to use. It's likely that soon she will be reciprocating the move.

Up on the Roof. One key to great foreplay is to attend to areas of the body that are often neglected. We'll find out more about these in upcoming chapters, but while kissing, you have an opportunity to stimulate one of them: the roof of the mouth. During a lingering French kiss, use your tongue to lavish attention on this erogenous zone, petting it with long strokes of your tongue and exerting gentle pressure along the inside rim. Be careful not to go as far as the soft palate though, as that can activate the gag reflex.

Teeth and Gums. If the above technique feels like too much tongue for your partner, try running your tongue over the teeth or gums, under his or her lips, or in the area where the tongue attaches to the floor of her mouth.

Switch Sides. Most couples assume the mouth-to-mouth orientation that feels most comfortable—that is, your face goes in one direction and your lover's goes in the other. For variation, try switching sides or kissing each other with your mouths precisely horizontal or perpendicular. And here's a great twist: Try kissing chin-to-forehead. This is a great prelude if one of you is heading downtown for some oral action!

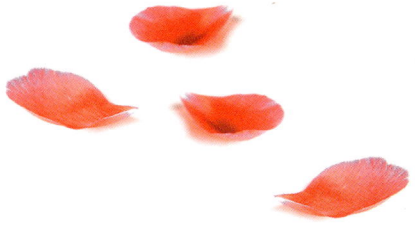

Helping Hands

Those variations should give your mouth a good start, but there's much more to kissing than what your faces are doing. Remember that erotic foreplay is a whole-body experience, and the more of yourselves you put into the process, the hotter it will get. What are your feet, pelvis, or torso up to while you are kissing? How about your hands? Hands, hands, hands . . . there is so much for them to explore, and so many ways to put them to use while kissing (see chapters 3 and 4 for lots more about erotic touch). Try some of these moves:

Circle of Love. A kiss is an embrace: Encircle your arms around your lover's waist and pull him in, applying enough pressure so that he feels encouraged that he is right where he belongs and that you are going nowhere.

Got Back? Use the flat of your hands to make gentle circles on her back, exploring her shoulder blades, waist, and each vertebra in turn. Vary your pressure from faint to light to insistent, but be careful not to press too hard on her backbone, as that can be painful for some people.

Let Your Fingers Do the Walking. Run one index finger up and down his spine ever so gently. There are so many nerve endings near the surface of the spinal column, you are sure to raise goose bumps with this one. Similarly, many people get an almost electrical charge out of the feeling of a finger run around the back of the waist, from one side to the other and back. Or try slipping a finger into the top of her crack, then run your hands down her backside and cup her ass in your hands. Booty delight!

More to Explore. Run your hands down the sides of his body, from under his armpits all the way past his waist and down his thighs. Linger over what feels good to your touch. Does he have a pair of little dimples, one above each buttock? Dip your pinky in each one and give it a swish.

Booty Call. After a gentle back massage, firmly cup her buttocks in your hands, feeling the beautiful globe shapes and their pillowy softness. Give them a little squeeze. While holding them, allow your pinky fingers to explore the crease underneath, between her buttocks and thighs. Your little fingers can creep tantalizingly toward her sex, but tease her by staying away from the prize . . . for now!

Beginner's Breaststroke. Although you don't want to focus too much on her breasts at this point, you can explore their sides and undersides. Try using the backs of your hands to do so, to vary the sensation. This is more of a light, brushing move than a squeezing one.

Hold On! Use your hands to punctuate what your mouth is doing: When you thrust your tongue deep into his mouth, use your hands to pull him in closer, either by grabbing his belt, holding his waist, or grabbing his ass. Turn up the heat by holding on tighter and harder and grinding your hips against his.

Get Ready for Your Close-up. Position yourself so you can press your pelvis to hers as you kiss. A firm hand on her lower back will help. Press your torsos together, or even weave your legs around one another's or wrap one leg around his waist, with your heel pressing into his buttocks—whatever it takes to meld your bodies into one. If you are standing, move her toward a wall and hold her in place by pressing your thigh between hers. You will probably get a moan out of this.

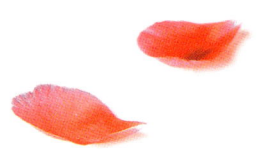

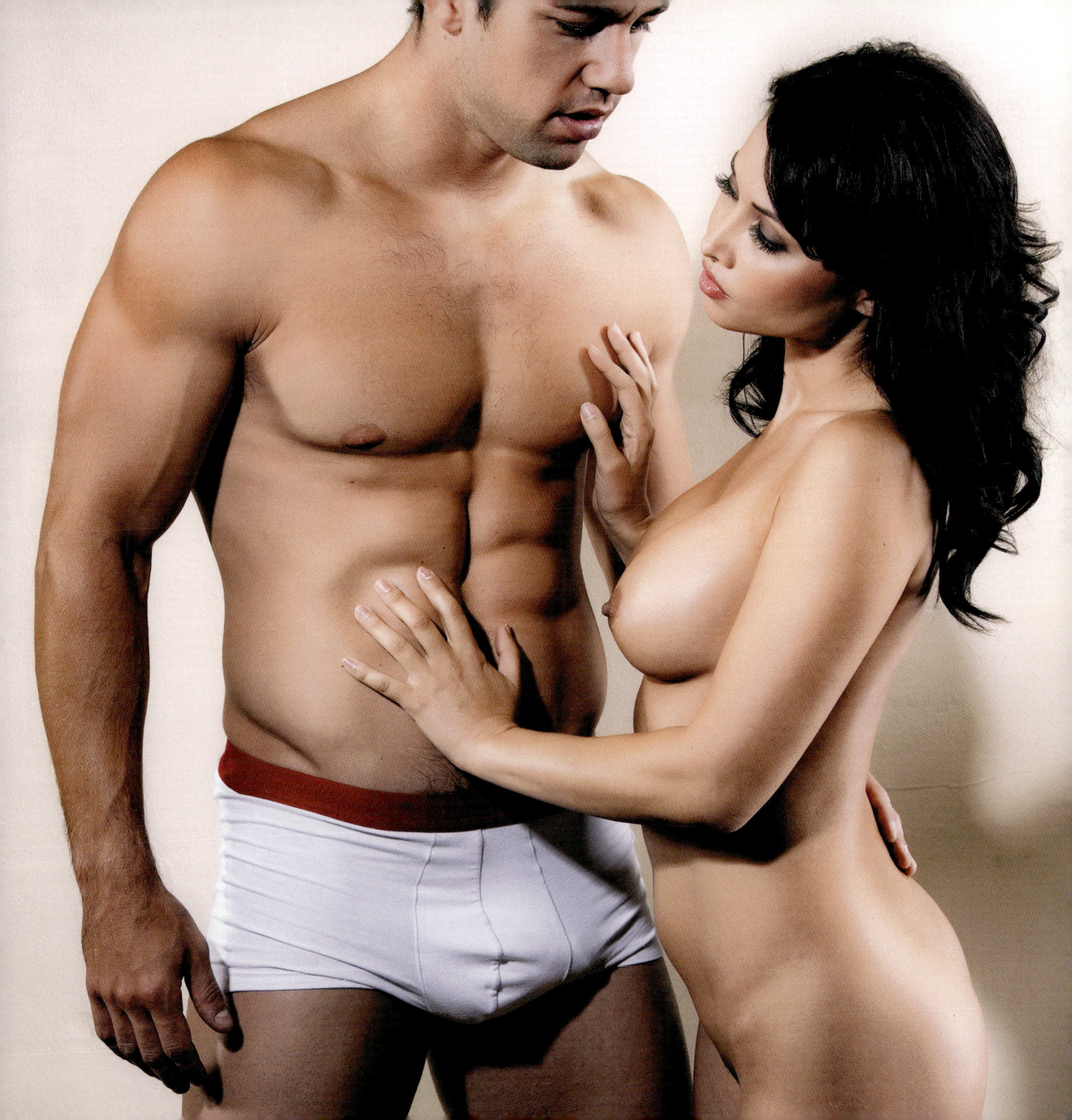

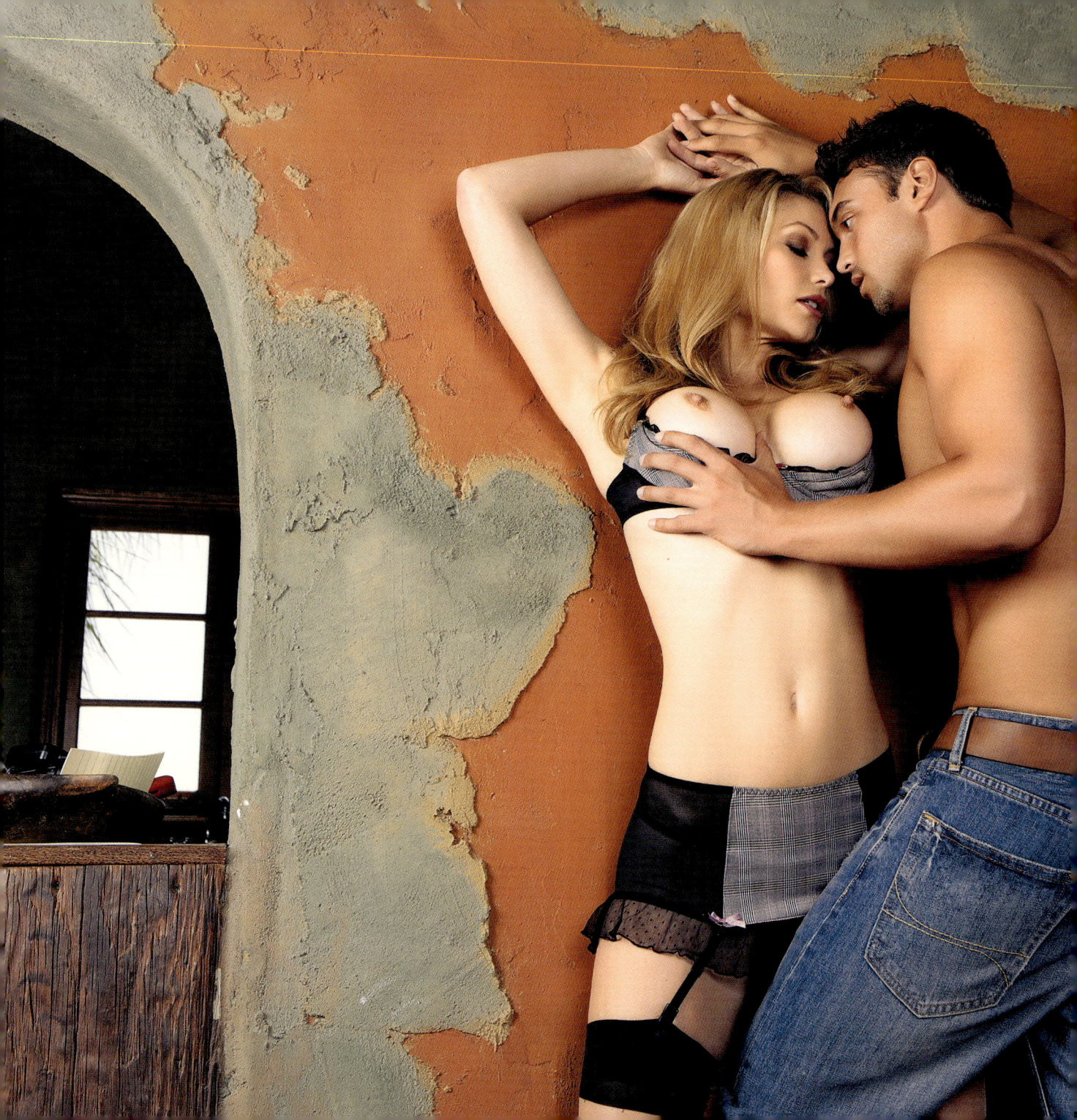

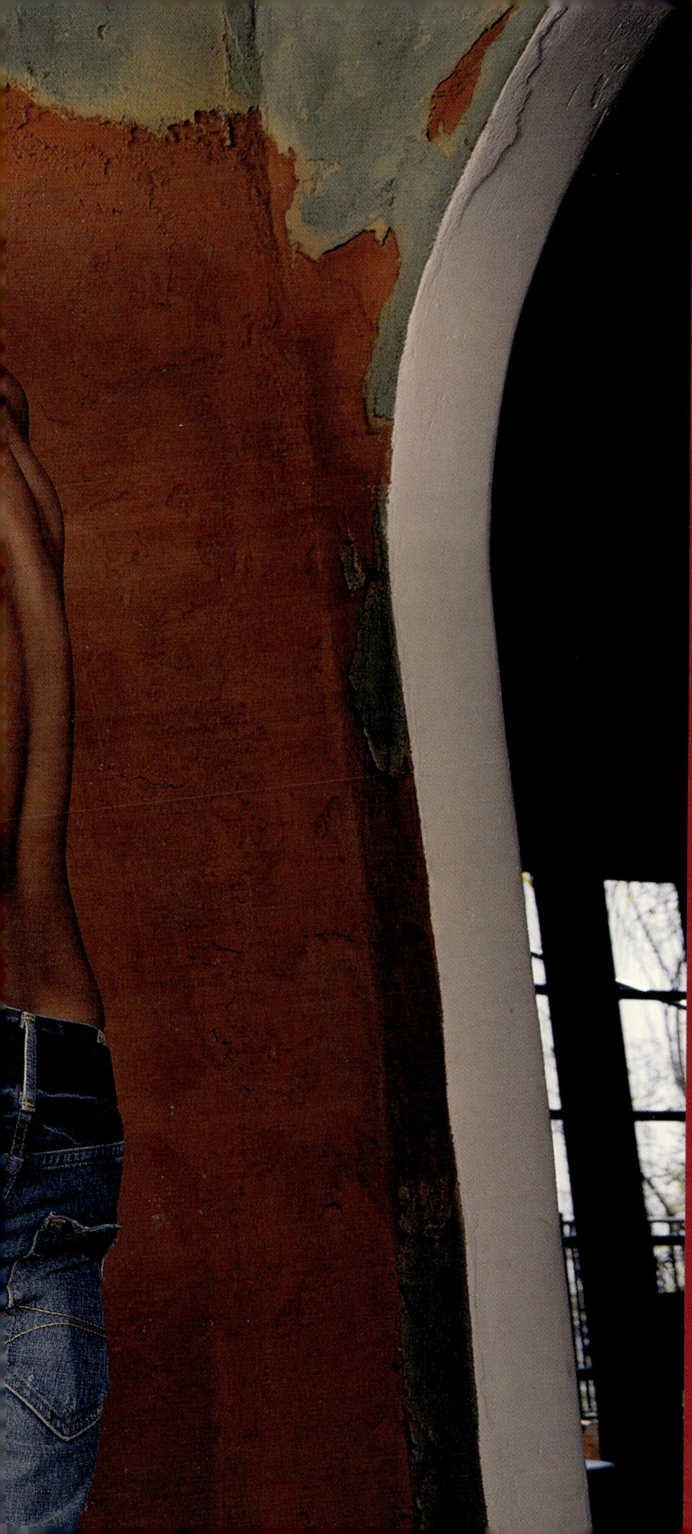

Face and Neck Time. Get creative: While you are kissing, stimulate the areas surrounding her mouth to enhance the sensual experience. Caress her neck, fondle her earlobes, drag your fingertips along the nape of her neck to give her a shiver, and stroke her cheeks.

Explore the Breasts. As your kisses heat up, try some more gentle exploration of her breasts as a hint of things to come. Cup them lightly, brush and circle her nipples or softly tweak them, or gently squeeze her breasts together.

Hands across the Universe. Use your imagination! In whatever position you're in—whether you're standing, sitting, or reclining—let your hands dance over whatever you can reach, probing, stroking, and teasing. Hand movement is great during a session of passionate kissing and will pave the way for lots more exploration later. If it seems appropriate, unbutton, unhook, or just plunge under those clothes—always remaining respectful of your partner's comfort level. I'll say it again: There is no need to rush, because lingering, teasing, and building anticipation is what great foreplay is all about.

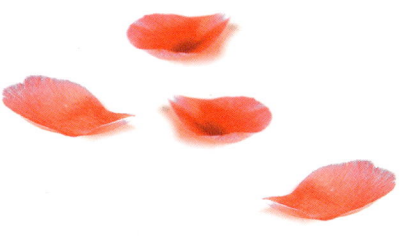

More with Mouths

According to an old song, "a kiss is just a kiss"—but we know it can be so much more. Going beyond mouth-on-mouth moves, your kisses can run all over your lover's anatomy during foreplay. Here are some suggestions to get you going:

Ring of Fire. Starting from her mouth, lightly kiss your way down to the base of her throat and then bestow a "necklace" of kisses around her throat. The neck and throat are filled with veins that bring blood to and from the brain, including the large carotid artery that runs near the ear. This area is ripe and responsive to shiver-inducing, exploratory kisses. While you're at it, find the hollow at the center of her throat and probe it with the tip of your tongue for a super sensation you will both enjoy. Find the pulse point behind her ear with your lips, and then feel her heart rate increase as you continue your kissing journey.

Handiwork. Take your lover's hand and gently work on each finger in turn, sucking on the tips. Remember: These are the hands that bring you exquisite pleasure. Smooch and nuzzle the back of his hand and along his forearm. Kiss his palms and supersensitive inner wrists (again, lots of blood flowing here), gradually moving up the silky-skinned inner arm to the crook of the elbow, and finally up to the armpit. If your lover is ticklish there, you might want to steer clear: A giggling fit could break the mood. But if you are getting a positive response, a few tongue flicks into the armpit can be dazzling, and you'll enjoy the sexy taste and scent as well. (There's nothing wrong with the musky aromas of the flesh, assuming you both follow the basic soap-and-water routine.)

Belly Dance. If you've opened up or removed your clothes, it might be time to explore your lover's beautiful midsection. Bisect his torso with your tongue tip, starting from the base of his throat and moving down to his belly button. Dive into that belly button and give it a wash with your tongue. Many people say that the feelings from a belly button probe extend straight into their core and emanate out to the tips of their fingers and toes. Don't neglect that area just below the belly button and above his pubic hair. Shower it with tiny, featherlight kisses, all while boldly stroking his thighs. He's sure to enjoy the contrast of soft and firm touching.

Thigh Master. The legs and feet are full of erogenous areas that respond to sweet kisses. Pay special attention to the soft inner thighs (so close to that prize!), the backs of the knees, grazing the shinbone, circling the ankles, and the instep of the foot. Shower these areas with light pecks or long brushes with slightly parted lips.

Toe-tal Pleasure. Which brings us to the toes—as delightfully suckable as the fingers are. Go to town on them: Toes and feet work hard all day, and a little attention to and appreciation of these appendages will be met with gratified sighs.

Flip Side. Don't forget to turn your lover over and explore his beautiful back and buttocks. Give his spine a tingle by suckling each vertebra and ending at his lower back. Then plant a few kisses on his butt cheeks to make him moan for more. Run your tongue around his lower back and into the top of his crack while you reach around and stroke his belly; alternatively, kiss, nibble, and nuzzle the back of his neck and earlobes while you run your hands up and down his front side.

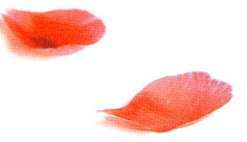

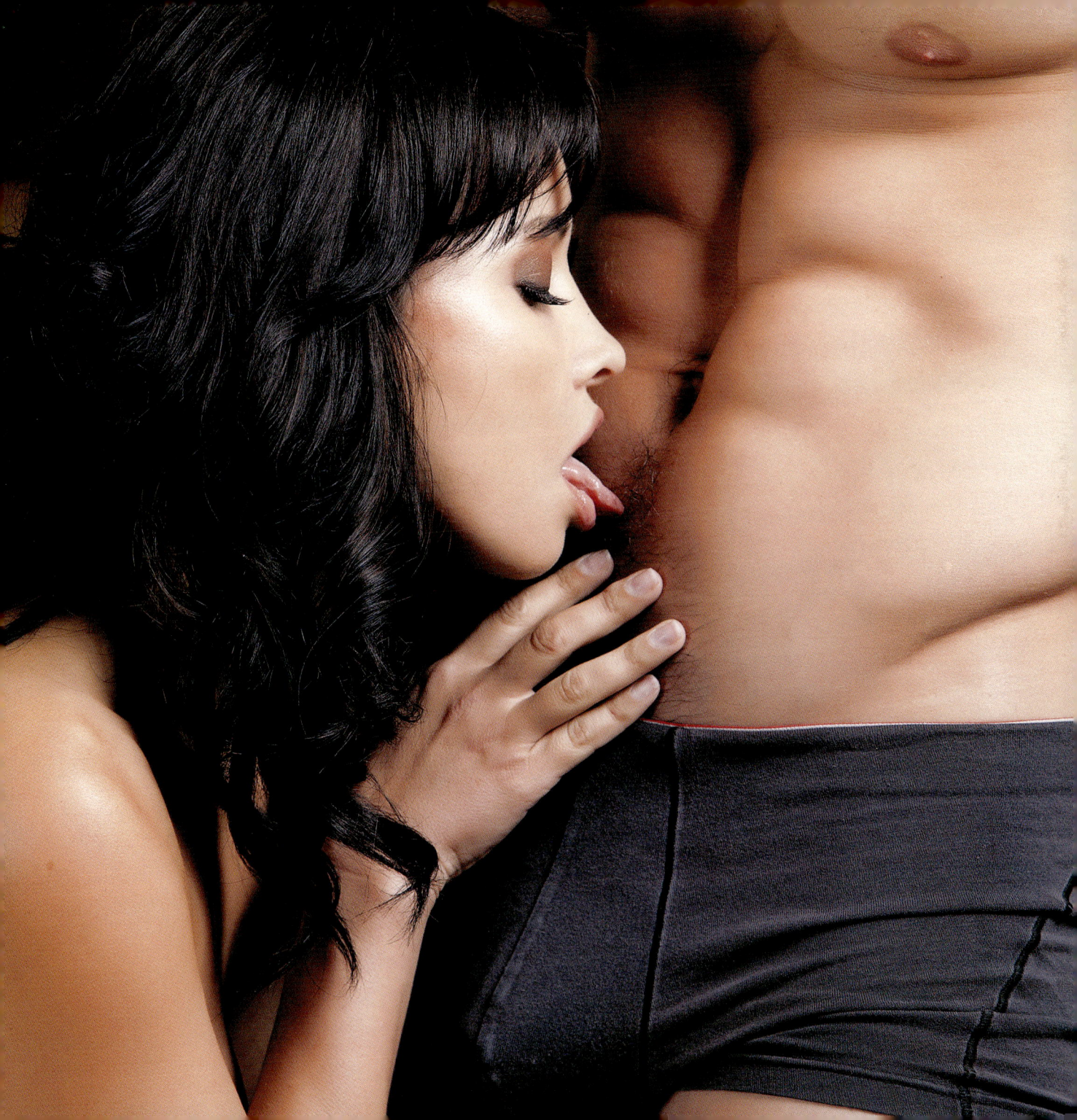

Tongue Tricks

Beyond conventional kissing and sucking, there is a variety of ways you can use your mouth on your lover:

A Little Nip. Change up your all-over kisses to include playful nipping and gentle biting. Watch how your lover responds. In general, men tend to like a little bit of force, including superficial biting and sucking. Women like it rough sometimes too, of course—but they tend to catch fire more readily with light body kisses employing an exquisitely gentle tongue and lips. It's better to make her urge you for more intensity than to overwhelm her with more than she can handle—especially at this stage of the game. Great nibbling spots include the neck, belly, inner thighs, buttocks, and even the nipples, if you find she enjoys that.

Grab a Bite. Speaking of sucking, you are surely familiar with the "love bite" (we used to call them "hickeys" as teenagers), in which you vigorously suction a small area of your partner's flesh with your mouth while also probing it with your tongue and teeth. This can certainly be erotic in its intensity—one of those moments when pleasure and pain collide for a few seconds—but beware of the telltale mark it leaves behind. Either let up before you create that scarlet blossom, or apply yourself to areas that are unlikely to be on view to others. (And if your lover asks you to stop, obey immediately, of course—as you would in all cases.) The classic love bite is on the super-erogenous upper neck, but there's no rule that says it can't be performed just above the breast, at the small of the waist, on the upper back, or elsewhere.

Lapping, flicking, stretching, swirling, nibbling, probing . . . be creative with your techniques as well as the focus of your attentions. And periodically return to that delicious mouth-on-mouth action that draws you together and urges you toward sexual fulfillment.

Take a Deep Breath

While we're on the subject of mouths, let's talk about the role of breathing in foreplay. Whether you're a dedicated yoga master or never really think about breathing except when you get winded while running for a bus, you should know that breath is much more than a physical need. Conscious breathing can enhance foreplay and sex, and it can be a useful tool in your arsenal of erotic techniques. Try these tips to imbue your foreplay with new life:

Breathe as One. While deep kissing, coordinate your breathing with your lover's and feel yourselves becoming deeply in tune. Share a few breaths by breathing into his mouth while he inhales, and then inhaling as he exhales. The reduced amount of oxygen in these shared breaths might even make you a bit lightheaded.

Heated Exchange. While kissing your partner's body, hold your mouth close to but slightly away from her skin and breathe out forcefully, as if you were fogging up a window. Then move to a new spot and do it again, creating little hot spots all over her body.

Ear Ecstasy. Hold your mouth close to his ear and breathe out gently. Instant chills! Alternate this with little ear kisses, lobe nibbles, and a tongue swirled around the inside of his ear and you'll have your lover in a trance of ecstasy.

Pants Are Tops. As you kiss and explore, keep your breathing deep and slow for awhile, then switch it up by doing some shallow panting. Then put some tone behind your breath so you let out a variety of sounds. Try breathing in through your nose and out through your mouth, then switch the order. Experiment with breath as part of foreplay, and you'll find that it helps whatever you are doing feel more organic and more satisfying. Breath is *life*, after all!

What Would Dr. Sex Say?

To perfect your foreplay techniques and reach those peaks of ecstasy, it is important to understand what, exactly, is happening to each of you during arousal—so here's a simple rundown of the biology behind the fireworks.

The word *foreplay* refers to the entire range of intimate psychological and physical acts that take place in an attempt to build up attraction and arousal and prepare your bodies for sexual intercourse (or other acts meant to bring you to orgasm). The goal, psychologically, is to lower your inhibitions and increase your emotional closeness. On the physical side, the point is to produce an erection in men and vaginal lubrication and expansion in women—all a prelude to the enjoyable sex to come.

For both sexes, the arousal or foreplay phase results in increases in the heart rate and breathing rate, and a rise in blood pressure. Almost all women experience erection of the nipples—and 60 percent of men do, too. Skin flushing (or vasocongestion) is common; some experts think there's a correlation between the degree of skin flushing and the intensity of the upcoming orgasm. (The redder the better, I guess you could say.)

Men, foreplay quickly leads to partial erection of your penis, but it is quite normal for this to wax and wane throughout the preliminaries. The testicles draw upward toward the perineum and the scrotum tends to tense and thicken—all in service of that impending erection.

Ladies, watch for your veins to become more visible and prominent, especially where your skin is thin (e.g., inner arms, breasts). Your breasts might even expand a little in size, and your nipples will elongate and become harder, as if begging for attention. Down below, your labia minora will probably grow in size and protrude from your labia majora, and your clitoris will become swollen with blood. (Who says women don't have erections?) You'll feel your vaginal juices start to flow, spurred on by the vasocongestion of the vaginal walls, which have now darkened in color and become smoother than normal. Something you may not detect is that your uterus is elevating—moving out of the way—and the inner two-thirds of your vagina is expanding up to 10 centimeters (almost 4 inches).

All of that said, arousal differs in each of us, so there is no normal response to sexual stimuli. The length of time it takes to become aroused varies greatly—not only from person to person, but also from occasion to occasion—as does the intensity of arousal. Each of us responds to different techniques at different speeds (and, of course, that's what this book is all about).

While we're on the subject of biology, think about this: Foreplay is actually one of the elements that separates humans from the animal kingdom. We are the only primates that do not have a *baculum*, or bone, in the male penis, making us the only ones who must become aroused to become erect and achieve penetration (and the obvious explanation for the term *boner*!). So . . . how important is foreplay? You could say it's keeping the human race going!

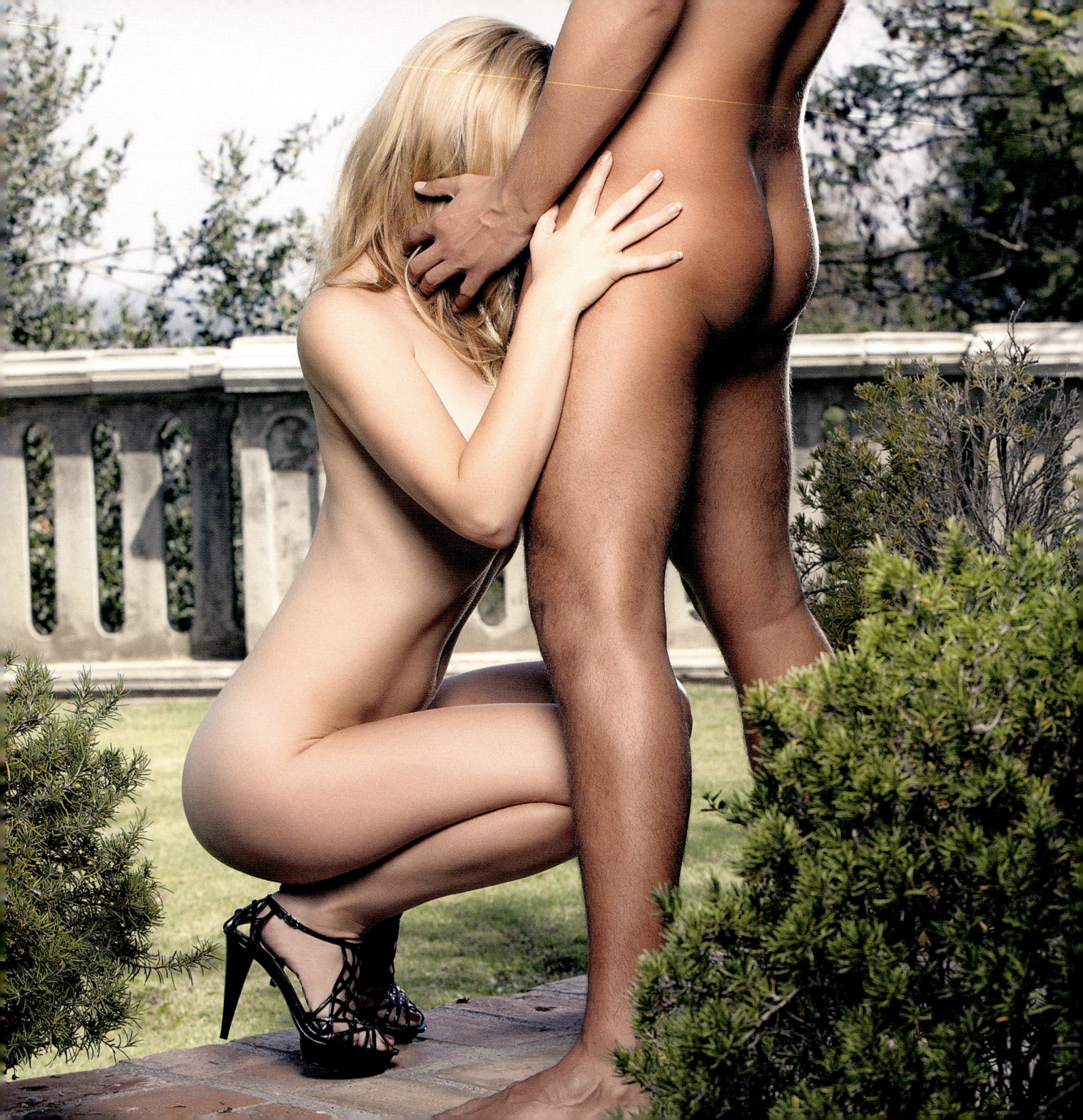

Hummm?

Humming as foreplay? Though it might sound silly, humming can be a natural vibrator. You've probably heard the slang term *hummer*, which refers to humming while performing fellatio (it works for cunnilingus as well!). But anything you do with your mouth can be enhanced by putting a little humming vibration into it. It might make you both laugh, but it feels great—and a little levity never hurts, either.

Kiss and Tell

Are you starting to see what an awesome means of foreplay your mouth can be? A great side benefit of all that smooching and licking, lapping and sucking is that kissing can be a kind of rehearsal for oral sex. Do to his tongue what you intend to do to his cock. As you are probing under her tongue with yours, imagine yourself prospecting for her G-spot. Your mouths are sensual orifices—sex organs, if you will—and when explored with skill and passion, they can be almost as potent and responsive as the organs down below.

Approach the kissing phase of foreplay with care and energy, and enjoy every minute of it as you awaken your mutual desire and bring your libidos into perfect alignment. Then, move on to the next level of the game: sensual touch.

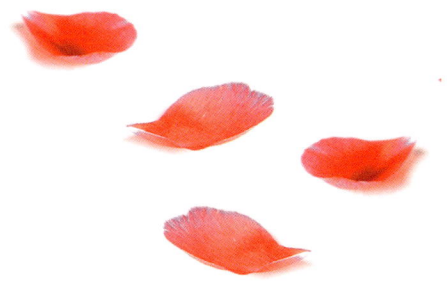

Hot to the Touch

The skin is a sex organ—your largest one—and it's just crying out to be stroked and attended to. It's filled with delicious nerve endings (and, by the way, women have even more of these than men do, which just might explain why we love tactile foreplay so much). From the time we were babies, touch has calmed us, warmed us, nurtured us, and made us feel happy, loved, and secure. It still does all of those things—and it prepares us for deeply satisfying sex.

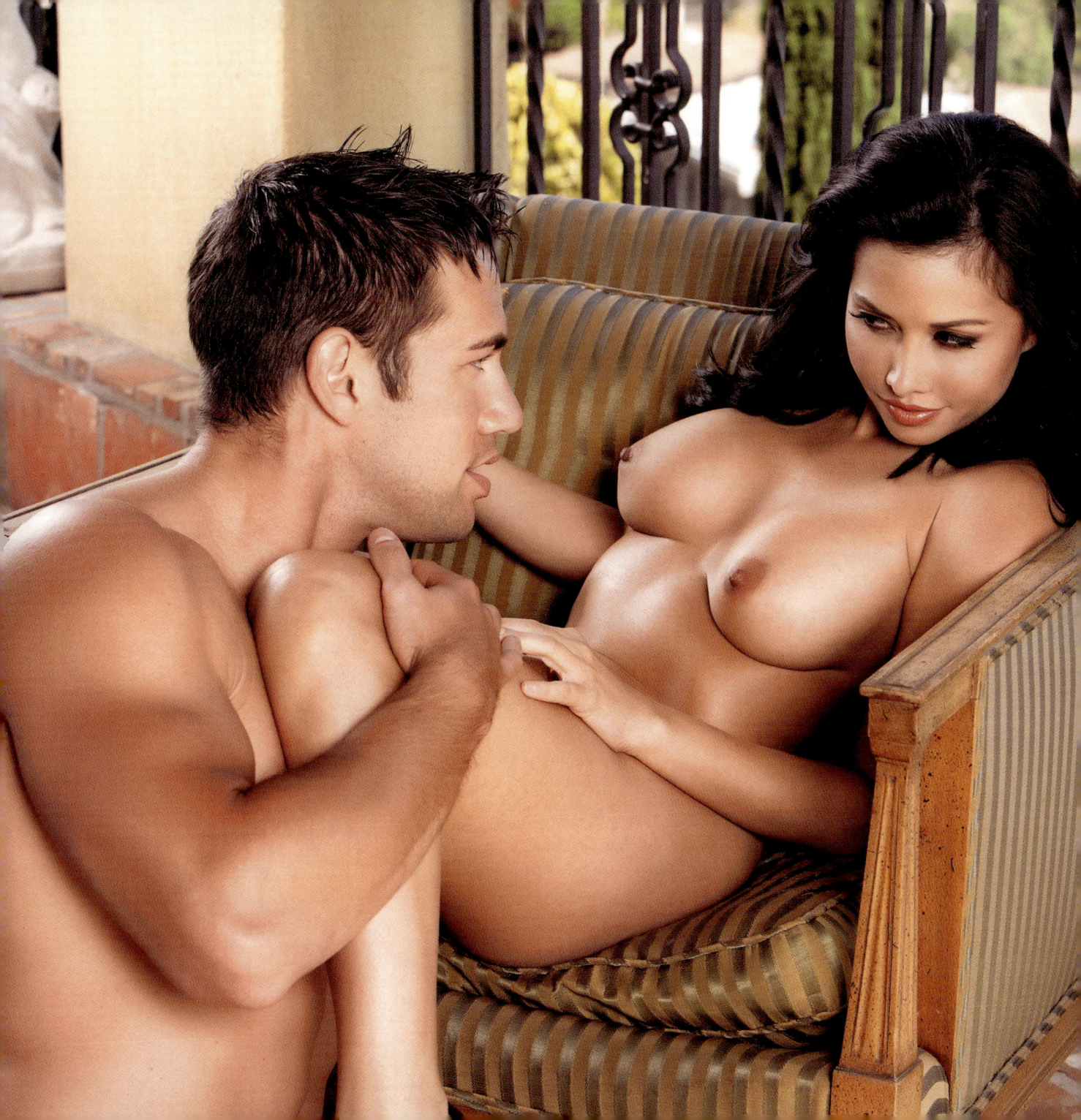

Much of what you do with your hands during foreplay probably seems instinctual. You're in the moment, going with the flow, doing what comes naturally. And that's great. (After all, sex isn't work; it's the highest form of fun!) But a little focus on exactly what you are doing with your hands and other moving parts can expand your foreplay vocabulary and introduce spicy new ways to please and tantalize your lover. For the sake of organization, we'll work our way down the body here, from top to toe (while leaving the genitals for a well-deserved chapter of their own). Of course, when you are putting these techniques into practice, there's no reason to follow a direct geographical route. You'll want to mix it up, be inventive, and surprise your partner. There are 45 miles (72 kilometers) of nerves throughout the average human body. With some creativity and a little thought, you can set them *all* tingling.

Here's something essential to keep in mind as you hone your foreplay skills: We tend to touch each other in ways that we ourselves would like to be touched—so be very aware of the specific ways your partner touches you, as these are probably the very techniques he or she would like *you* to use. Does she tend to use long, featherlight strokes up and down your body? Try the very same thing on her, and you are bound to get an ecstatic response. Does he like to knead your shoulders with his thumbs and fingertips? Give him a massage in return and feel his temperature rise. Turnabout is *more* than fair play in foreplay.

The flip side of this is useful, too. Is there something you wish your partner would do during foreplay? Show him! If a lighter, more tickly touch turns you on, demonstrate it on him and he is likely to follow your lead. If you wish she would give your scalp a delicious rubbing, let your own fingers show her the way. Of course this isn't the only means of communicating your likes and dislikes. A heart-to-heart talk is sometimes called for, and we've got some helpful tips for that later in the book. But if you are wondering what your partner wants, relax and pay attention to what he or she is doing to *you*. Mirroring that is a great place to start.

One more note about massage: While they aren't strictly necessary, oils and lotions have lubricating qualities that make massage much more enjoyable and fun for both parties. Lubrication isn't just for sex; it happens to be a great foreplay helper, too.

Different Forms of Touch

Before we start our tactile journey, let's pause to explore the different touch techniques at our fingertips. As you explore your partner's fabulous anatomy, remember that variety—in both style and intensity—keeps things spicy. Here are some basic techniques to try, and feel free to invent your own:

Tapping or drumming your fingers feels particularly nice on the firmer parts of your lover's body, including the back, waist, and legs. Try tapping your fingers lightly on her sex as a prelude to more intense probing.

Twirling and swirling your fingertips on the breasts or buttocks feels fantastic. You can also swirl in a circle around her nipples, or twirl your fingertips around the curve of her shoulder.

Finger-walking down the abdomen, thighs, back, or buttocks will slow down the action a little for a tantalizing break. Walking your fingertips close to erogenous zones then quickly backing off can help build the anticipation.

Firmly rub to provide a blissful massage to the arms and hands or calves and feet, as well as the back.

Grip and release for a nice variation when you are attending to your lover's limbs and extremities, as well as her waist and (gently!) her neck. Try gently gripping and releasing her ass or shoulders, too.

Touch and disappear. For this one, have your partner close his eyes so your next touch will be a surprise. Use any of the touch techniques, and switch them up.

Long, cascading strokes can be delicious anywhere. Use both hands, fingers slightly splayed, and vary the speed from a fast, whooshing move to a slow, sensual stroke. This is especially nice if he's lying on top of you; use your entire forearm to stroke his back from the shoulders to the top of his thighs.

Use two hands for two different forms of touch. If you are coordinated, try different techniques simultaneously, one with each hand. Try a smooth stroke on her thigh while you grip and release her breast.

Light slapping, tapping, and smacking can be delightful for some people, especially on the ass, thighs, or even breasts. Try gently slapping his erect penis and see what happens.

Gentle or deep massage, using your palms, the heels of your hands, and even your forearms and elbows, is a supremely sensual form of foreplay. Use massage liberally, paying close attention to the areas where your lover responds most intensely. Back, front, limbs, neck—and don't forget the head—all warm up to a lovely massage.

Fingernail scrapes or digs are a spicy variation that can make him tingle. Try this on his scalp, back, or thighs.

Featherlight tickling is another way to change it up by slowing down the action. Get feathery on her breasts, behind, and inner thighs.

Tongue touching means using the tip of your tongue like a finger to explore your lover. Ears are particularly fond of tongues, as are nipples, inner thighs, and the top of the crack.

Gently pushing or twisting can also be very sensual. Try pushing her breast taut, then teasing her nipple, or very gently twisting the skin of her waist between your thumb and forefinger.

Get forearms, elbows, fists, and even toes into the act, and use your imagination to come up with an endless variety of techniques to drive each other wild.

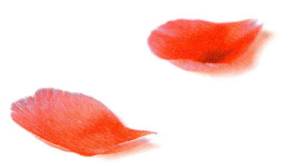

Head, Neck, and Shoulders

Oh, the head is a glorious place to begin a conversation about touch! Your skull is so much more than a helmet to protect your brain. It includes your face, sinuses, ears, eyes, scalp, and, at the base of your skull, the all-important brain stem that connects your cerebrum and spinal cord. The neck and shoulders are the workhorses of the body, and for that reason, they are the most prone to the buildup of tension throughout the day. Great foreplay can release all of that tension, sweep those cares aside, and pave the way for super sex. Here are some specific ideas to get you started:

Think a Head. Give your partner a soothing head rub by using just the tips of your fingers in a firm, circular motion. Keep the circles small, though, so you won't pull the hair. After ten seconds or so, reposition your hands and keep going. Don't leave out the forehead. Try anchoring your thumbs at the base of the skull, on either side of the nape of the neck, while you work the back of the head with your fingers. You should see the tension drain from your lover's face in short order.

Hair Today. You may think there's no feeling in the hair, but the scalp and head are so sensitive, and hair is so sensual, that playing with hair is a great addition to your foreplay arsenal. Stroke it, twist it, get lost in it, braid it, grab handfuls of it and pull gently—or hard, depending on the response you get. If it is sufficiently long, you can hold your lover "captive" by the hair—a great beginning if you are working up to some playful bondage (see chapter 6 for more on that).

All Ears. Ear play is great foreplay. Starting at the top and moving down toward the earlobe, use your thumb and forefinger to gently massage the ear. Give a little extra attention to the area in the middle, close to the opening of the ear canal and the little lip closest to the cheek—but don't stick your fingers into the ear holes. Massage both ears simultaneously or take turns, and be sure to adjust the pressure based on your lover's response. Alternate this with some of those hot ear kisses we talked about in chapter 2, and watch things catch fire.

Eyes on the Prize. Working on the eyes takes finesse, as they are very sensitive, but a little attention there is a wonderful romantic gesture. Alternate light eyelid kisses with gentle thumb-stroking just under the eyebrows and across them to show your lover how attentive you can be to every detail. The bridge of the nose is a wonderful place to linger as well: Gently rub the tension away with your thumb and forefinger (this is especially good if your partner usually wears glasses).

Face Time. Working on your lover's face is a wonderful time to stare into her eyes—and eye contact is an essential element of great foreplay. Place your hands on her cheeks and gently hold her face. Brush her lips with your fingers, then very lightly work your thumbs and fingertips down the sides of her throat to get some chills going. The pressure points in the neck and throat make for some delicious sensations there.

Sweet Stranglehold. During foreplay you are establishing trust and closeness, so a gesture that might seem threatening in another context can be perfectly welcome and appropriate. Gently placing your hands around your lover's throat in a position that resembles choking can actually make him feel safe and cared for, especially when you use your fingers to rub out the tension in the back of his neck.

Soft Shoulders. Some of our largest and most active muscles can be found in the shoulders, and they are literally responsible for all of the heavy lifting we do every day. If you want to get serious about your lover's shoulders, have her lie face down on the couch or bed and straddle her on your knees for good leverage. Start close to the neck, kneading her shoulders with your full hands and fingers. Her reaction will help set the intensity level. Hold the balls of her shoulders in your palms and squeeze; use your thumbs on the upper back, feeling for tension spots and gently massaging them out. The winglike shoulder blades will love the sensual attention; place your palms over them and squeeze. Alternate massage with light and feathery strokes. (If you and your partner find yourselves particularly intrigued by massage, there are many classes available for couples. Check out both your local fitness center or adult education center.)

Arms and Hands, Front and Back

We continue our journey down the body with the torso, front and back. This, our core, provides a rich playground for sensual touch of all kinds:

Loving Arms. To wake up your partner's arms, use both hands, fingers spread wide, to stroke the length of each arm, one at a time, from shoulder to fingertip in a swooshing motion. Alternate arms and vary the speed of your strokes. Turn your lover's arms so that the undersides are facing up and give her some slow, whisper-light strokes on the supersensitive wrists and forearms. Try blowing on them as well. In the places where you can see the blood vessels, there are loads of throbbing nerves right near the surface, begging to be stimulated.

Handicraft. The hands are worth serious attention because they contain pressure points that will send sensations reverberating through the rest of the body. Massage each finger and thumb slowly and lovingly, using a firm touch. Use your thumbs to vigorously work on the palms—you can even get your chin into the action. But apply a gentler touch to the backs of the hands, where the bones and blood vessels are close to the surface. Tightly encircle the wrists with your thumb and forefinger and squeeze as you rotate them under your touch. Try pulling each finger in turn to give your partner a lovely little stretch. Shower the back of his hand with featherlight kisses, then slip your tongue into the tiny crevices between the fingers as if you were flicking your tongue into his crack.

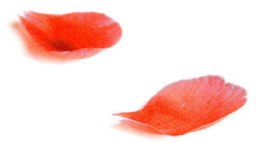

Breast Friends for Life. Your lover's breasts are the lovely, erotic centerpiece of foreplay—or "second base," as some like to say. You could spend an hour on her breasts alone, using your hands, your mouth, and lots of imagination. The important thing is that you remember how exquisitely sensitive they are and treat them accordingly. Stroke them gently and lovingly, give them a playful squeeze, lap the nipple with the flat of your tongue and then circle it with the tip—but never maul or manhandle them, no matter how turned on you get from seeing and touching them. Gently suck on each nipple, while probing and circling it with your tongue. Try cupping your lover's breasts from below to feel their weight, suppleness, and round shape. Bury your face between them and taste the salt of her sweat. Give the nipples a little pinch, gently roll them between your forefinger and thumb, and explore them with your palms and fingers. Can you feel them get hard? For a really subtle move, just hold your warm palm above her nipple, without touching it, and try to get her nipple to "reach" for you just from the heat of your hand.

Back and Forth. If your lover enjoys having you stimulate one breast and nipple at a time, imagine her level of arousal when you go back and forth between them! Try gently pushing the breasts toward each other, then use your tongue to suck, lick, and softly bite each nipple, moving quickly back and forth between them. This flurry of activity is sure to melt her core.

Watch and Learn. Now try this supersexy move: Ask your lover to fondle her own breasts while you watch. Not only will you both get very turned on, you will learn something about how she likes to be touched. Make a mental note of every little move she makes and replicate each one when you get your hands on her.

Men Have Them, Too. Did you know that men's chests and nipples are erogenous as well? Sensitivity varies from guy to guy, but trust me: Don't ignore him in that area. Stroke his chest with the flat of your hand, pausing to feel his nipples under your palms. Circle your palms over his nipples. Can you feel them harden the same way yours do? Now give them a lick; give them a gentle suckle. Take turns teasing each nipple with your mouth. You'll know from his reaction whether you have hit gold. If he is loving the chest action, don't stop!

Back Bliss. As for the flip side, backs may not be as directly erogenous as fronts—but there are lots of ways to touch and caress the back that your mate is sure to enjoy. Consult all of those touch techniques discussed earlier and liberally change up your style, from long swooshing strokes to pinches, love taps, and deep knuckle-kneading. The lower back, in particular, is a highly erogenous zone, so give it extra-special care, applying both gentle and firmer touches.

Back Massage. Remember: Relatively few people pay for sex, but lots pay handsomely for massages! And here's an added plus: Giving someone a vigorous back massage is great exercise. You'll be burning calories while you are gearing up for great sex. Try the straddle position described earlier; the spoon position with you behind your mate, tucked in close at the knees; or the reach-around, where you are face to face so you can kiss and coo while you work on one another's B sides. Let your hands explore each other's backs using a light, teasing touch alternated with firm kneading. The waist is a particularly nice place to linger, and don't forget to work your hands up and down your partner's sides for some chills and thrills. Don't neglect the

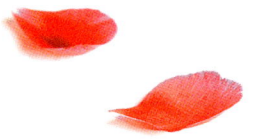

Watch and Learn

Ask your lover to fondle her breasts and make a mental note of every little move she makes. Not only will you both get really turned on, but also you'll learn how she likes to be touched.

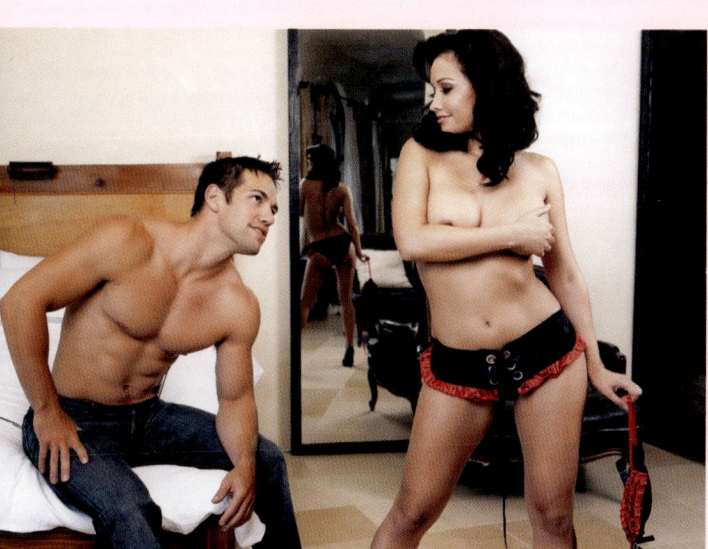
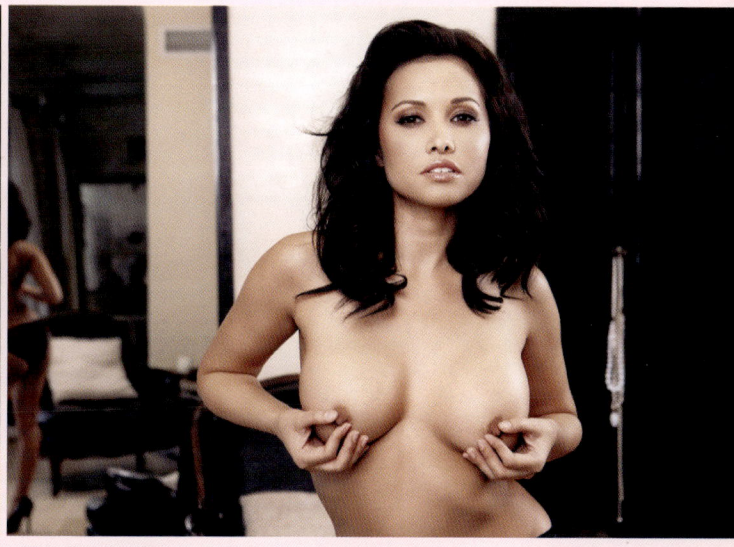
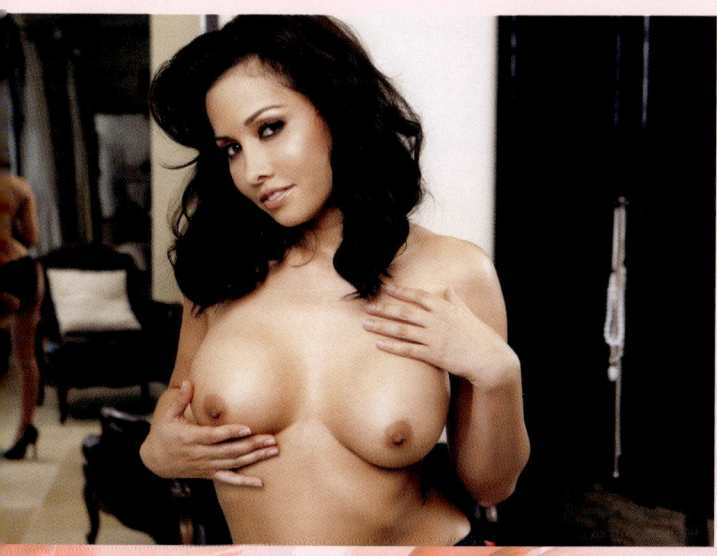
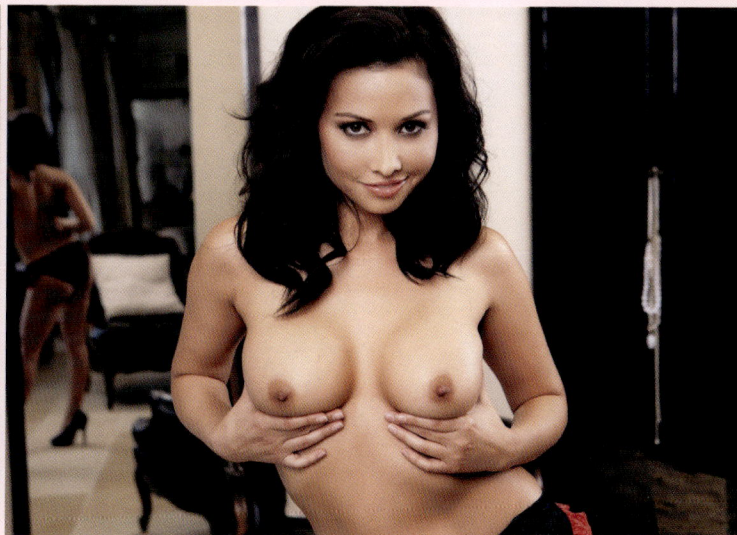

upper arms. Smooth your hands down your lover's shoulders and gently grip and release the upper arms, biceps, and forearms. The back is a great place to get your fingernails into the action, too. You don't want to draw blood, but sometimes a little bit of light clawing can raise goose bumps. Alternate long vertical caresses up and down the back, accompanied by little squeezes. Take care of the supersensitive backbone by lovingly feeling each vertebra, from top to bottom. Professional masseuses often use their forearms and elbows on their clients' backs, and this can be a fun way for you to play. Get your whole body into the act for a greater sense of closeness and lots of intriguing sensations for both of you.

Tummy Tickler. And here we are at the stomach, the lovely runway to paradise, where things start to get really exciting. Some of us are self-conscious about our stomachs, but with some loving care and encouragement, you and your lover can make one another feel supersexy and desirable. Use your hands and mouth liberally on the tummy, lingering over the beautiful line straight down the middle, from chest to belly button. Gentle laps, licks, and kisses, alternating with light finger massage, will get the blood flowing. Whether you are using your tongue or your fingertip, don't forget to explore the belly button itself—a very erotic and tingly little organ in its own right. Grasp your lover on either side of his waist while you cover his abdomen with delicious kisses. He'll be moaning for you to go lower, but take your own sweet time and bring him to a full boil before even thinking of diving for the prize.

Backside, Legs, and Down to the Toes

Bottoms Up. Time to pay homage to your lover's beautiful buttocks, another large-muscled, hardworking area of the body that deserves a little tenderness—and that goes for boys *and* girls. Start by grasping the globes of her ass and pulling her close to you. Gently caress her buttocks, allowing your fingers to graze the crease between them and the lovely folds where they meet her legs. Want to try a few little pinches or smacks? Go for it, but be sensitive to her reaction. Turn her over and just look at that beautiful behind! (Foreplay is visual too, you know.) Hold it, squeeze it, kiss it, tap it . . . let her know you treasure it. Knead her ass as if it were her breast, tease her ass crack, and then go a little deeper, gently caressing the area between her anus and vagina. Lick her gently at the top of the buttocks while you reach around with one hand and slowly stroke her pubis—soon she'll be moaning for more!

Endgames. Kiss *his* ass? Absolutely! All of the actions described above go for you, too, ladies. Let him know that his manly behind is delightful to look at and a pleasure to hold, tease, smooch, and fondle. Try caressing the area under his testicles and right up the crack of his ass. As you do this, be aware of his response; if he seems game, break out the lube and press into his anus a bit with your fingertip. (There is a lot more about penetrating touch coming up.)

Leg Love. Long strokes with firm fingers up and down the legs can be exquisitely pleasurable—these limbs so rarely receive any intimate attention. Take turns massaging and stroking one another's legs, paying special attention to the inner thighs and the backs of the knees, which are very sensitive areas, just like the forearms and inner elbows. The Achilles tendon, which is most prominent just behind the ankle, can always use some gentle massage to relieve the tension that builds as it propels us through our daily life. As elsewhere, there's more to taking care of the legs than simple massage. Try light scratches with your nails, cup the knees and then release, and remember those back-of-the-knee licks and kisses.

Foot Fancy. Finally, the feet. And really, is there anything more pleasurable than some serious foot play? Women who get spa pedicures know the secret: The warm whirlpool action and lubed-up foot massage are the best parts! Work on your lover's feet one at a time, focusing on every single toe and in between each one. Make a fist and use it to rub the bottoms of his feet. Use your thumbs to press out each toe pad (underneath, where each toe meets the foot) and squeeze his insteps and the balls of his heels. Press your four fingers between his five toes, close your hand, and squeeze. This may all seem a bit remote from sex, but I assure you it isn't. The pressure points you'll be stimulating will resonate throughout his body, right up through his core. And, again, toes love sucking, insteps love kissing, and feet love all-over squeezing. Try squeezing each foot between your thighs to provide a new sensation for both of you.

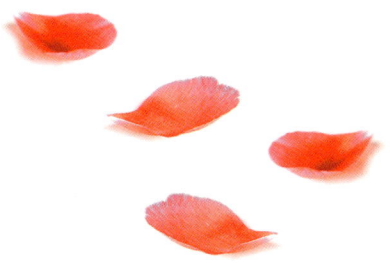

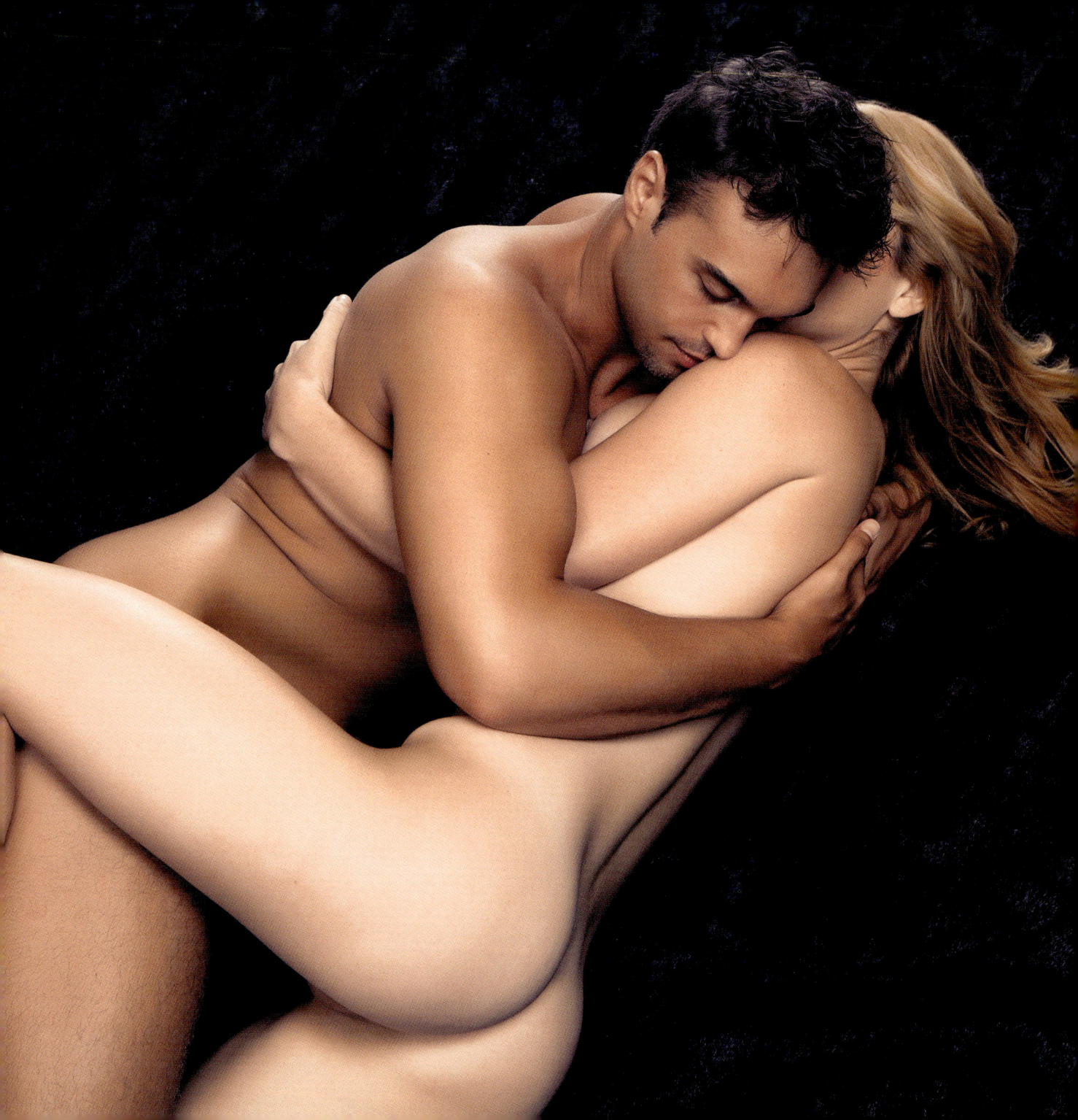

Good All Over

While we're on the subject of touch, let's not forget the all-important hug. Hugs can be wholesome, yes, but they can also be highly sensual and are an important part of the close bond you are establishing in foreplay. Hug each other often and at length, wonderful full-body hugs where you make as many points of contact as possible and move continually to create lovely mutual pressure. Try hugs standing, sitting, and lying down; try them facing each other and one behind the other. Here's a fun one: Lie on your backs and turn your faces toward each other, your hips close together, and wrap your legs around one another's waist. A leg hug! (Hand-holding is a nice addition to this one.) Now stand back to back, interlock arms, and hug yourselves. The buttock-to-buttock pressure feels great, doesn't it? Next, lie on your sides, face to face, with your arms wrapped tightly around each other and your chins resting on each other's shoulder. This is a great way to relax and feel close.

Think of more variations. The sweet, snug embrace that a hug provides, that surrounding pressure, is a beautiful lead-in to the hug of sexual penetration.

Clothing as Constraint

As you explore your lover with your hands and mouth, keep in mind that leaving bits of clothing on (as opposed to always being completely naked) can be quite sexy. Doing so can make you feel as if you are stealing a feel or returning to younger days, when you didn't dare take off all your clothes, no matter how badly you wanted to. Touching through clothes is divine, and will leave you both damp with desire—but don't worry, those wet spots dry.

Instead of racing to undress her, caress her breasts through her blouse and bra; stroke her labia through her silk panties, then push them aside and touch her directly to make her gasp.

Ladies, your man will love every second that you stroke his (no doubt expanding) cock through his pants before you unzip him and let it out. Staying dressed or semidressed can make foreplay feel a little bit naughty—and naughty can be nice.

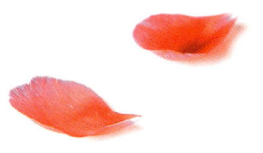

Slo-Mo, Tip to Toe

Think of yourself as Columbus and your lover's body as a vast, mysterious new world. It's time to chart every inch. Try tracing the outline of your lover's body from the top of her head down to the tips of her toes. You can do this with a fingertip, your nose, a string of kisses—just go slowly, lingering over and appreciating each beautiful inch of her. If her impulse is to move, you might want to tell her to hold very still instead (or employ some kind of gentle restraint). This kind of slow and deliberate attention will cause the tension to build and the sexual juices to flow, even if what you are doing is subtle and quite innocent. And, too, just as she is feeling the sensation of your fingers (or nose, or kisses) playing over her body, your fingers are experiencing exquisite feelings as well, and sending them right to the pleasure center of your brain. Never skimp on exploring each other by hand, but when you keep it simple, you are doing less and feeling more. Speaking of . . .

The Almost Touch

Did you know that you can give a whole massage without even *touching* your lover? It's true. Your hands radiate energy and warmth, which can be felt by your lover even without your touch. Ask him to close his eyes. Hold your hands *near* his ody, getting as close as you can without touching him. Make concentric circles with your hands, or long stroking motions, or rapid back-and-forth waves. This near-touching just might drive him mad with desire for your touch—but ask him to concentrate and really feel the energy between you.

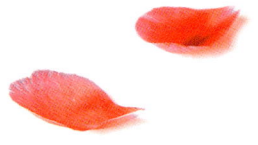

To Come, or Not to Come?

With apologies to Shakespeare: To come or not to come? That is the question. Considering the variety of pleasure techniques covered in this book, you must be wondering about the issue of coming during foreplay.

There's no right or wrong answer to this question. Lots of women are multiorgasmic and have no qualms about coming whenever they feel so moved. (Some come exclusively during foreplay and focus on their mates during penetration. Others come before and during—and maybe even after!) For men, multiple orgasms can be elusive or time-consuming, so some work hard to hold back on coming until later in the game.

It's not up to me to tell you when foreplay turns into sex—but my feeling is that female orgasms during genital foreplay are deeply gratifying to both partners, and no impediment to the great sex that will follow. There's no particular reason for a woman to hold back an orgasm unless she wants to, and no reason she can't come over and over during a session of creative and generous lovemaking. But watch out, gentlemen: Once you've unleashed your lover's ability to achieve multiple orgasms, there will be no going back! (Do keep in mind that, while a rest or refractory period between orgasms isn't always necessary for women, they can be hypersensitive after an orgasm, and thus functionally needing a rest of their own.)

Ladies, if you and your man both like the idea of making him come during foreplay (watching him spew his sperm can be sooooooo sexy), then be sure to give him enough time and love afterward to recover and get ready to go again before you resume lovemaking. The refractory period in men, that necessary intermission between performances, varies tremendously in length, based on age and other factors. According to some studies, eighteen-year-olds can be ready to go again in fifteen minutes, while seventy-year-olds might need as long as twenty hours. The average time for most men tends to be about half an hour.

If you *don't* want to come during foreplay, however, here are some ways you can help each other hold back until you are ready to let loose:

Know the Signs. To help your partner hold back his or her orgasm (or even to encourage it), you have to know when it's coming. Watch for the telltale signs: an intensifying of the sounds he or she makes (moaning, giving instructions); writhing or, in some women's cases, going completely still; a retraction of the woman's clitoris under its hood; or the further stiffening of the man's penis and pulling up of the scrotum. If you are going to try to stop an orgasm, don't wait until it has started!

Desensitize. Lots of men know this trick already. If you are concerned about coming too soon, wear a condom. The slight desensitizing effect that the layer of latex has might help you hold back until you are good and ready.

Ice. An ice cube to the neck or back can be the perfect distraction from orgasm, but don't make this a complete surprise or you risk the wrath of a chilled and startled partner. This technique should only be used as a sexual aid, not a practical joke.

Stop. If you sense your partner is moving toward climax too quickly, slow down what you are doing—or just stop completely. Wait for the feeling to pass, then resume. Sexual response can be like a wave: Sometimes it's best to just float over the top of it and wait for the perfect curl to bring you in.

Part II:
Moreplay

Going for the Gold: Fun Down Under

Now that we are waist-deep in foreplay (as it were) and have explored the many ways we can tease and awaken one another from tip to toe, it's time to get down to the delightful business of the genitals. Perhaps you bought this book thinking that it would focus exclusively down there and have been wondering when we'd finally get to the point. By now I'm sure you understand that foreplay is a rich, varied, all-over (and all-inner) endeavor. But still, there comes a time when the panties and briefs come off and the preliminaries to sex begin in earnest.

Many elements of foreplay transcend gender: What's good for the goose is good for the gander. So in most chapters of this book, we've mixed it up for mutual satisfaction and fun. But as we go south of the equator, our anatomies diverge and so do the techniques we can apply to drive our partners to delightful distraction. For the sake of genital foreplay, let's focus on the ladies first (attention, gentlemen), and then turn our attention to the men (your turn to learn, ladies).

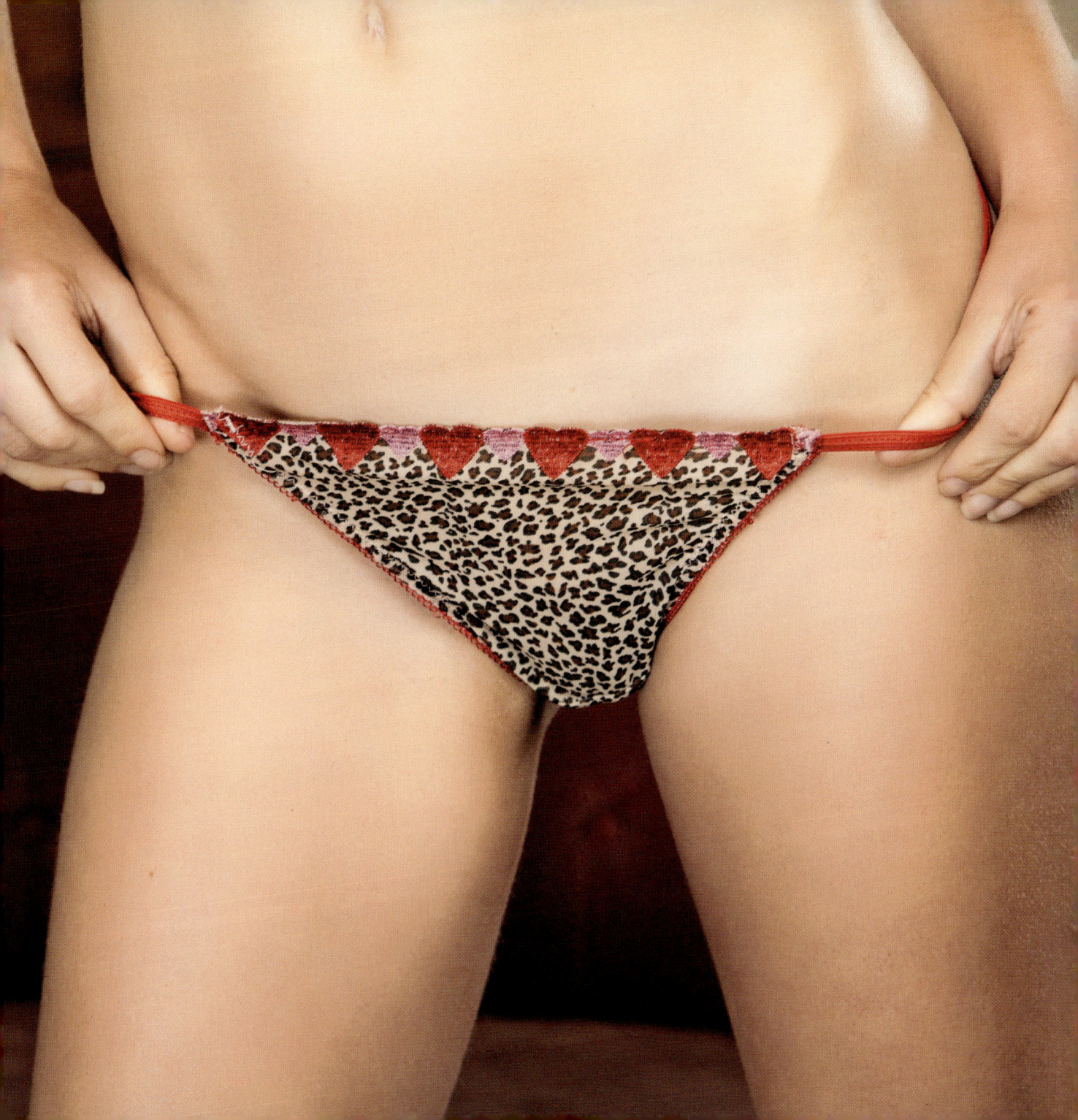

Just for Men: Your Pleasure Guide to *Her*

Things are getting hot and heavy. You've flirted and teased, massaged and necked, sweet-talked and petted. You've taken your time, fully focused your attention on one another, and gotten yourselves in tune. Your penis is probably semierect (at least), and she is beginning to drip with luscious lubrication. Before you plunge into oral sex or intercourse, though, here are some stimulating diversions to spice it all up even more. By the time you are done with her, she'll be begging for action!

But first, a visual guide to girls, so you understand all the moving parts:

You might already know your way around down there pretty well, but it is always good to know the official names for these parts. While we're on that subject, the word *vulva* refers to those parts that are outside the body—most of what is relevant to foreplay.

The labia majora and labia minora are the two sets of folded skin, large and small (*labia* means "lips," and that's what they look and feel like), surrounding the opening to the reproductive tract. The clitoris (remember how it's pronounced: not like the mouthwash Lavoris—but with the emphasis on the first syllable) is a small nub of extremely sensitive tissue—the equivalent of your penis, and every bit as responsive—protected by the prepuce, a very necessary little "hoodie" that veils it from sensations that might be too intense. And the vaginal opening is that freeway to paradise that you've been headed toward all along. (We'll talk about exploring it with your hands in the ultimate foreplay gambit.)

Now that you have the lay of the land, it's time to explore your lover's sweet spots in ways that will really turn her on. As always, mix it up, multitask, take meaningful pauses, and pay close attention to her responses so you can fine-tune your techniques accordingly:

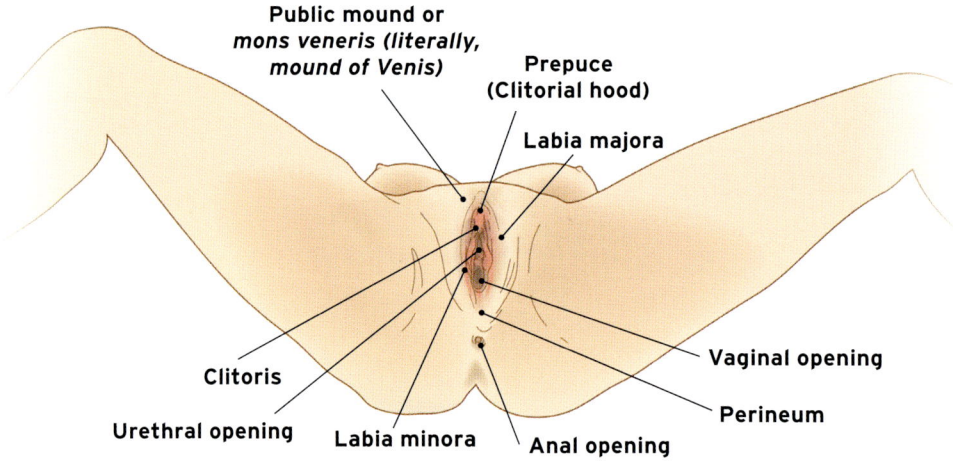

Public mound or mons veneris (literally, mound of Venis)

Prepuce (Clitorial hood)

Labia majora

Clitoris

Urethral opening

Labia minora

Anal opening

Vaginal opening

Perineum

Look, Don't Leap. Before you lay a finger on your lover, take a minute to admire her. (Even by candlelight or a dim lamp, you'll be able to see plenty.) Sit her down on the bed or sofa and slip off any of her clothing that remains. Gently spread her legs, caressing her thighs as you do, and look at her clitoris, labia, and vaginal opening. Some women are a little self-conscious about how they look down there, possibly because they haven't spent enough time admiring *themselves.* You can bolster your lover's confidence greatly with some loving looks, a gasp or two, and compliments galore. Make sure to lock eyes with your lover often during foreplay; maybe you can even get a gasp from her with your eyes alone.

Climb Every Mountain. When it is time to touch, aim high at first. That lovely exterior pubic mound, with the prominent pubic bone standing sentry at its base, is like the delta of her deep, fertile river. Stroke this area lightly with your fingertips. Now, place your full hand over her beautiful mound. Instead of aiming your fingers *toward* your lover's vaginal opening (where they will very likely end up), start by placing the heel of your hand at the bone and your fingers splayed upward toward her belly. Hold her that way for a minute, feeling her warmth emanating into your hand. Increase and decrease the pressure of your hand in a sort of stationary massage or squeezing action. Then gradually stroke downward with your fingers again, ending at the pubic bone (which brings you very close to that little hood covering her precious clitoris). Vary your strokes with a few gentle pinches of the skin around this area or gentle tugs on her pubic hair. You should be getting some positive feedback as your mate's inner and outer sex organs start preparing in earnest for what (and who) is to come.

Seams Heavenly. Explore the crease between the thighs and the vulva, running from the front of her legs down toward her backside. This crease is deliciously *close* to her sex, but still slightly removed from it and a tantalizing place to tease, as it is filled with nerve endings. Run your index fingers along these borders, but make sure to stop if she's too ticklish there. Repeat this slowly, at least eight or ten times, until she begs you to move on to more.

Lips Over Lightly. At this point, your lover's outer and inner labia are probably getting swollen, darkening in color because they are engorged with blood, and becoming more sensitive than usual. So when you first lay hands on her lips, use a whisper-soft touch and light stroking movements with the very tips of your fingers. Many women find that long, slow strokes of the labia majora drive them as wild as any penetrating touch could ever do. (One way that women differ profoundly from men is that in the area of erotic touch, lighter is often sexier; for men, a more vigorous approach is the touch of choice—especially when moving toward a climax. In general, men have thicker skin and fewer nerve endings, which explains why they need more manhandling.) Change up your speed and the length of your strokes to determine what she likes best: Try shorter bursts or little pokes of the labia, which have become wonderfully spongy for you; squeeze the lips together as if you are closing her "mouth" and massage them together; then spread them apart with your thumb and fingers. Concentrate on the outer lips for awhile, allowing her the exciting anticipation of the deeper touch to come. Blow on those inner lips to create extra chills. Use a circular motion starting by stroking the crease area, then moving to the outer vulva, and finally the inner vulva; end by moving your tongue in a circular fashion around her clitoris. In general, circular motions are a big turn-on for women; there's something about having each area touched in turn, all the while feeling your touch moving closer and closer to *that* spot.

Change It Up. There's no need to stay in the same body position (if you still are). Sit your lover on your lap sideways, stretch out face to face, kneel between her legs on the bed as she lies back, sit behind her and allow her to recline into your chest so you can nibble on her neck as you explore—whatever gives you comfortable access and makes both of you feel connected and close.

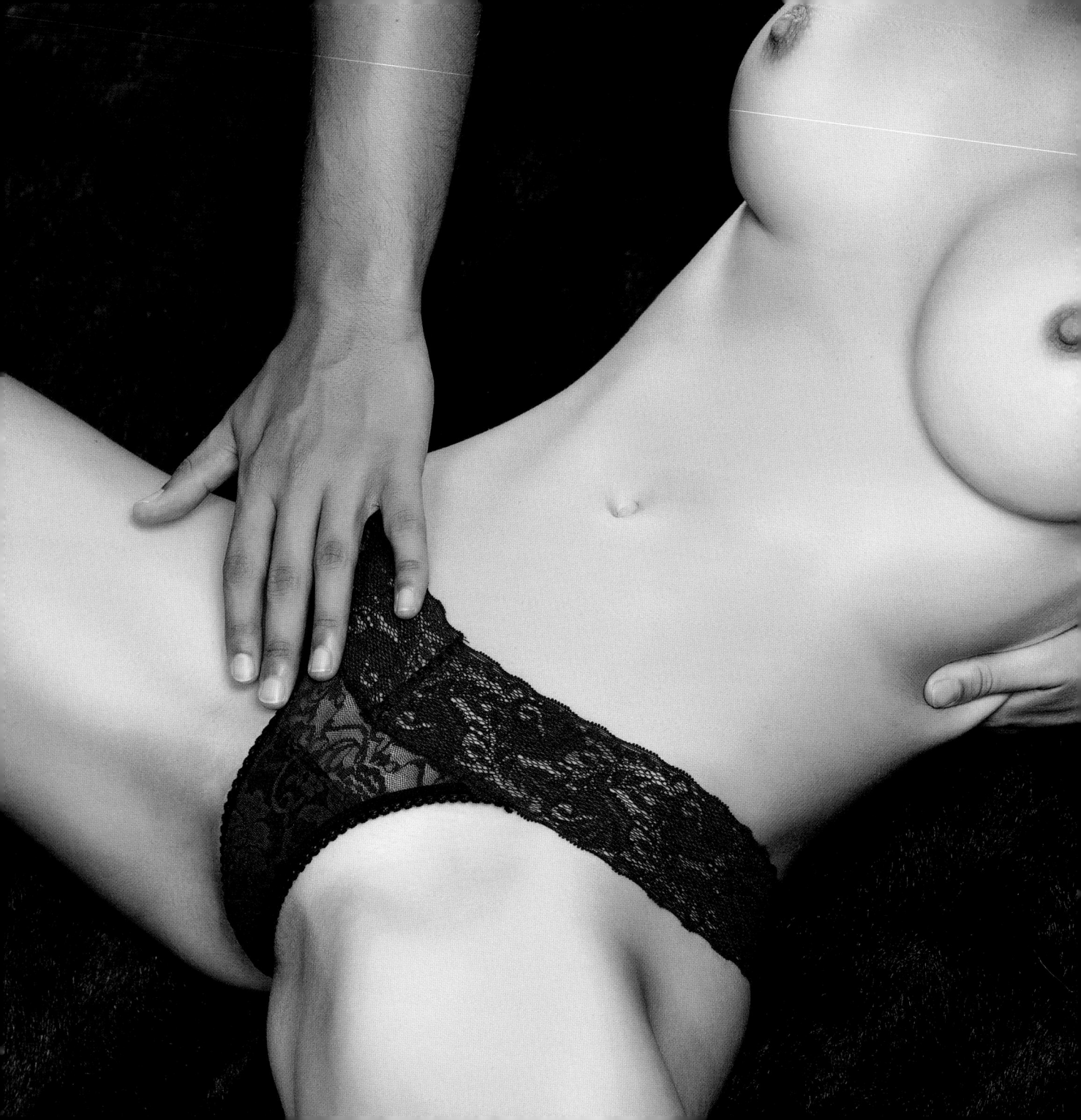

You've Got Rhythm. Here's a similarity between ladies and gentlemen: Repetition is key to building toward climax. So . . . although variety is spicy and changing up your touch techniques keeps the action exciting, you don't want to be too chaotic or disjointed in your movements when you get to the genital area. When you find a stroke your lover responds to or an area that makes her moan, stick with it or stay there for awhile, allowing her to get lost in the rhythm of your touch. (This is just as important—if not more so—during cunnilingus and intercourse as during foreplay.) Repetition builds erotic momentum, and that leads to smashing orgasms!

Slippery When Wet. As you move your attention from the outer to the inner labia, you'll find her getting slicker—but maybe not slick enough. Every woman lubricates differently, and as we age, we lubricate less. So use your own saliva or keep some light lube handy to smooth over your fingers as you begin to explore your lover's vulva more deeply. Start probing the inner lips surrounding her vaginal opening using your fingertips or the first knuckles of your index fingers, but hold back as you move toward the top, near the clitoris. Vary your approach, facing your hand toward her back sometimes, then toward her belly other times. Use a light touch, but make it progressively firmer, relying on your partner to guide you with her responses. Both of you should be getting pretty worked up at this point—but there are a few more places it might be nice to explore before you allow yourselves to move on from foreplay to...play.

Clitoris Clues. You've probably been wondering about the mysteries of the clitoris ever since you first heard about sex in any explicit detail. That little pleasure bud nestled under the prepuce is so intensely sensitive in most women that touching it directly can be painful. Always lubricate when you explore this area with your partner and discover with her whether she prefers the direct approach or a more indirect one, where you stimulate and agitate the flesh around and over the clitoris rather than the organ itself. Try massaging and pressing on the pubic mound, prepuce, and the lips on either side. Tap, stroke, gently squeeze, jiggle . . . and vary the pace. A rapid but soft, vibrating, back-and-forth movement of your fingers or palms against various points on the surrounding vulva can make her clitoris sing. All of these moves can work directly on the clitoris, too, if that's what she enjoys. When it comes to female pleasure, the clitoris is ground zero.

Inside Story. When it's time to try a little penetrating touch on your lover, you might be able to put the lube aside if her juices are flowing. At this point her vaginal canal is expanding to prepare for your entry. Start by slipping one finger inside, with your palm facing up, a little way at first, and then deeper; when you are in up to your large knuckle, wiggle your finger in a beckoning sign, as if you are saying "come here." Guess what? You've probably nailed her G-spot! It's not a myth, and it wasn't so hard to find, was it? Caress it and feel her squirm with delight. Twist and turn your finger as she "hugs" it with her vagina; slide it in deeper and then out again, finding a rhythm she likes; wag it back and forth as if saying "Tsk, tsk." Slide out your finger and, in one smooth motion, run it up her vulva and around her clitoris, then back into her opening. Not only will she writhe with pleasure, but you'll lubricate her clitoris for the next move: With your finger still inside her, use your thumb to tease and stimulate the clit, pressing the hood between your thumb and the finger inside and massaging. Then lift your thumb and quickly insert your finger even deeper in. Is she gasping?

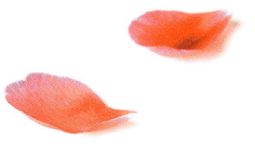

All In. When you've explored the one-finger possibilities to your mutual satisfaction (all the while using your other hand all over her body, especially against her sweet behind), you might want to try slipping your thumb, two fingers, or even three fingers inside her, depending on her reaction. (When she is pressing her pelvis into your hand, you can pretty much assume she is asking for more; if she's pulling away, it is time to fine-tune your movements or replenish your lube. Finger-fucking may sound old-fashioned, but its effectiveness has stood the test of time. With several fingers inside her, you can experiment with new moves: Spread your fingers slightly and contract, rub them together, cross them, twist and turn them. And while one hand is occupied inside your lover, use the other to fondle a breast, tweak her nipple, smooth her hair, tickle her back, or run your tongue around her clitoris. Continuously attend to the vulva, rather than focusing solely on her vaginal canal; be creative—but always thoughtful and aware of her reactions.

To the Backside. Assuming you are both comfortable with a trip to your lover's anal area, this can be a rewarding arena for foreplay. Start by moving your fingers up her perineum (the soft tissue between her vaginal opening and her anus). On both men and women, this area can be exquisitely sensitive, since it is directly connected to all of that spongy erectile tissue you've been stimulating—and because it is probably starved for attention. The perineum can handle a fair amount of pressure, so bear down a little, using her natural lubrication or some extra lube to help you slide your fingers smoothly toward her anus. Move your fingers back and forth over the length of her perineum, enjoying its slickness and proximity to all of her welcoming orifices.

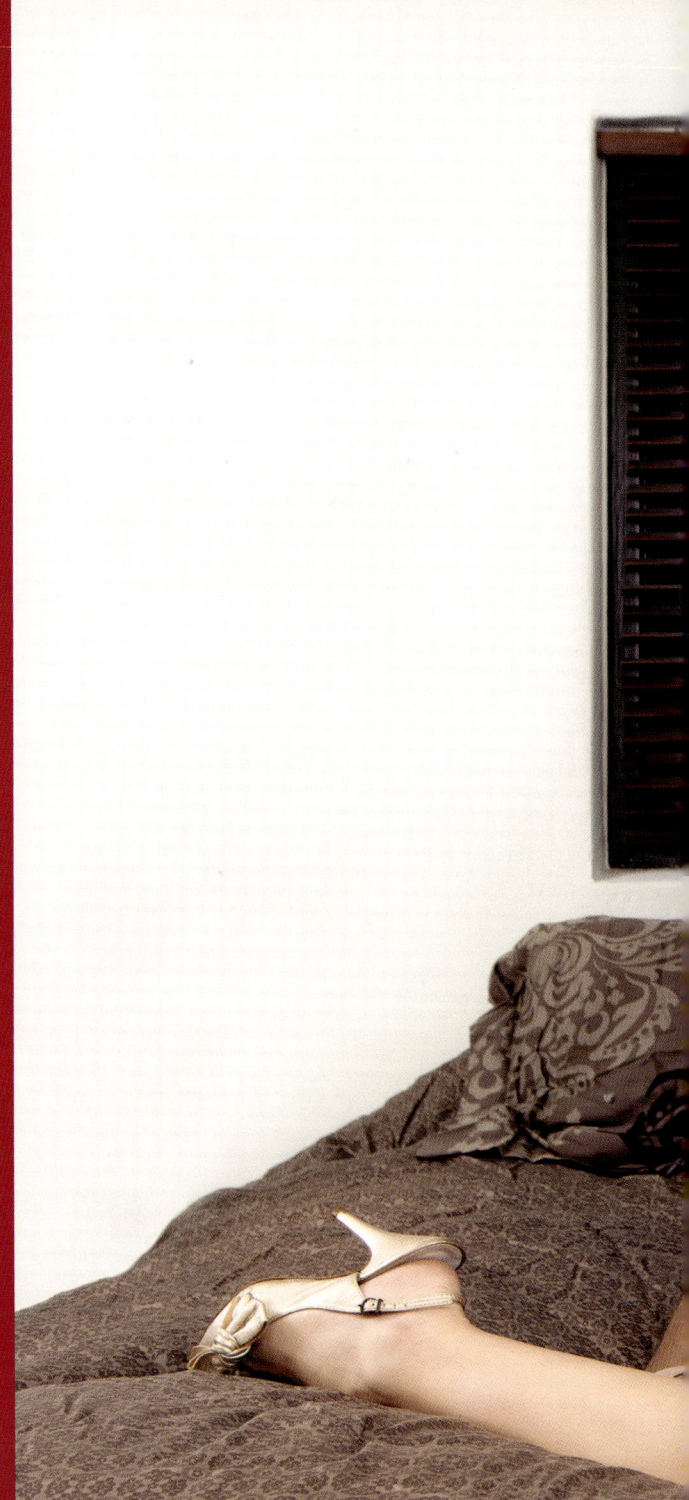

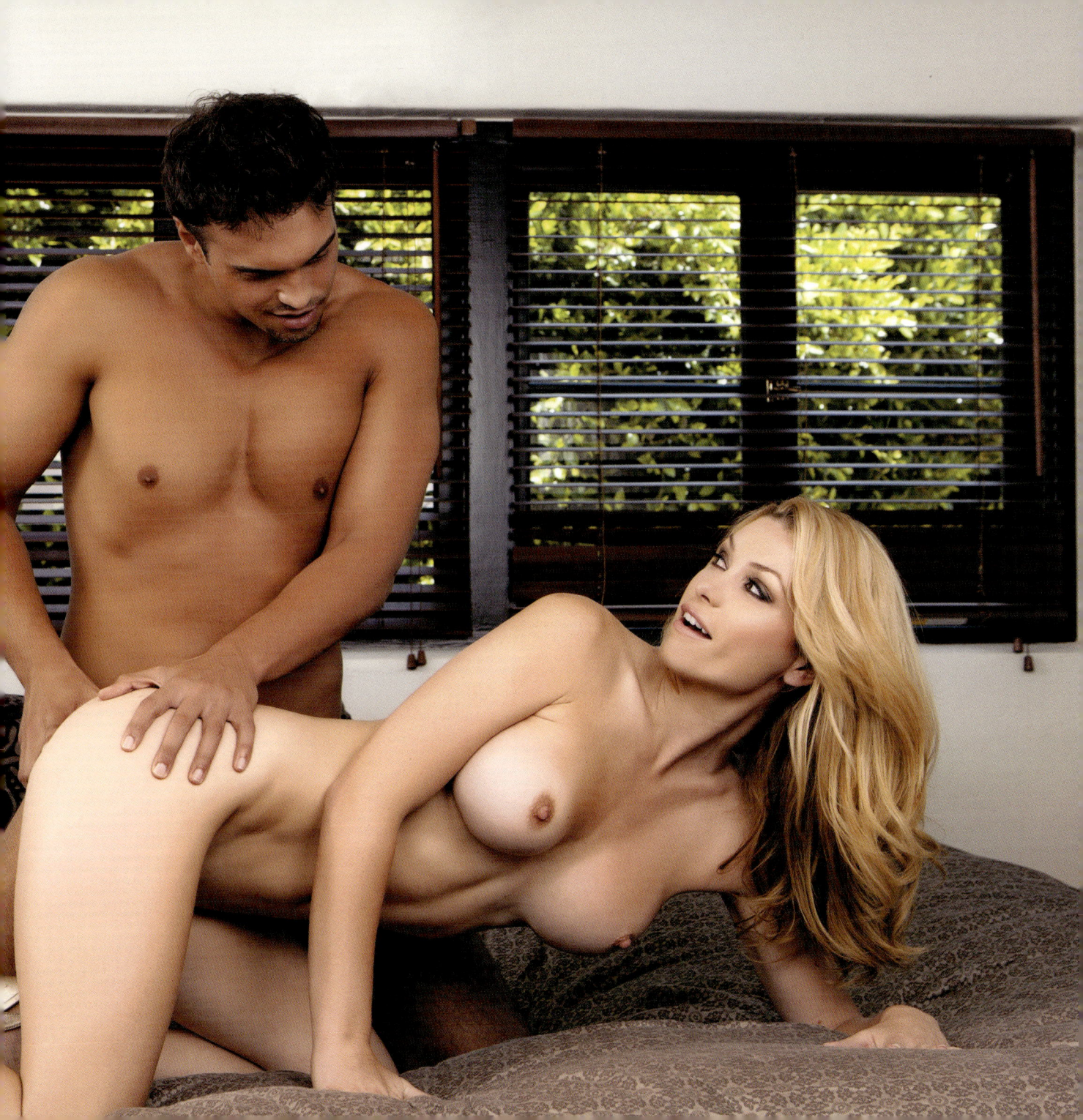

Anal Made Easy. Anal play is a similar experience for men or women (though men sometimes have bigger issues about penetration—and you'll hear more about the role of the prostate gland soon). If you are communicating well with your partner, you should know whether she is comfortable with you going there—and if she is, you are both in for some fun. Position her on her belly, either flat or with her buttocks in the air; on her side, with you either behind or in front of her; over your knees, as if ready for a spanking; or in any accessible and comfortable position. Make sure that everything is clean and well-lubricated. If you'd feel more comfortable wearing latex over your finger, by all means don a finger condom (usually called a finger cot and found at both sex shops and medical supply stores) and lube it up. Start by running a finger around her anal opening, teasing it and helping it relax. This is a delightful area to explore, pink and puckered like a little mouth, ringed with powerful muscles and delightfully flexible. Because we are used to the sensation of material moving *out* of our anus rather than in, you may find she tenses up when you come calling at this doorway. That's natural. Give her some time, whisper encouragement in her ear, continue fondling her, and she should soon relax and open herself to you.

Venturing Inside. When you feel she is ready, gently insert one slippery fingertip—just a very little way at first. Is she relaxing more, or trying to squeeze you out? Stay still for a few seconds until she opens for you, then twist your fingertip a bit, always paying attention to her response. Cradle and stroke her with your other hand, whether she is facedown or face-up, so she feels safe and cared for. (If she is facedown, a hand under her belly will be calming and may come in handy when it is time to exert more pressure; if she has her butt in the air, fondle her breasts; if she is sitting on your lap, hold her around her waist.) If all is going well, gradually deepen your penetration and increase your movement. In everything sexual—but in anal play, particularly—there is no right or wrong way to feel or progress; it's a matter of mutual comfort and satisfaction. If you find yourselves becoming interested in anal sex in general, there are some very good books devoted exclusively to the subject. But even if it's not your cup of tea, a little stimulation back there can heat things up in brand new ways.

Intro to Oral: Men's Division

I said in the beginning of this book that we weren't going to delve too deeply into oral sex, since that is a bit over the line from foreplay (and whole books have been devoted to it—rightly so!). But since we're on the subject of female genital stimulation, it would seem like an oversight not to include some surefire oral techniques along with the manual ones. Ready to dive in?

A Few Laps. Your tongue can be every bit as agile and playful as your fingers and hands, so use it with confidence and creativity. Start by lapping her labia and the entire vulva area from anus to pubis with long, luxurious strokes. Flatten your tongue out as much as you can and cover as much surface area with one lap as possible. Work back to front, getting a slow, steady rhythm going and gauge her reaction; some women love this more than almost anything. Gradually increase the pace. You might just cause an orgasm with this one move.

The Runaround. Make your tongue rigid and use the tip to explore the folds and creases around her labia. Circle her vaginal opening. Bend her legs back so her anus is exposed and run the tip of your tongue up toward her anus, roaming and playing there before going back to the labia, flicking them gently with your tongue.

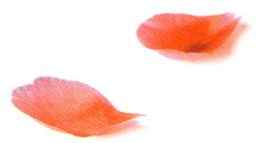

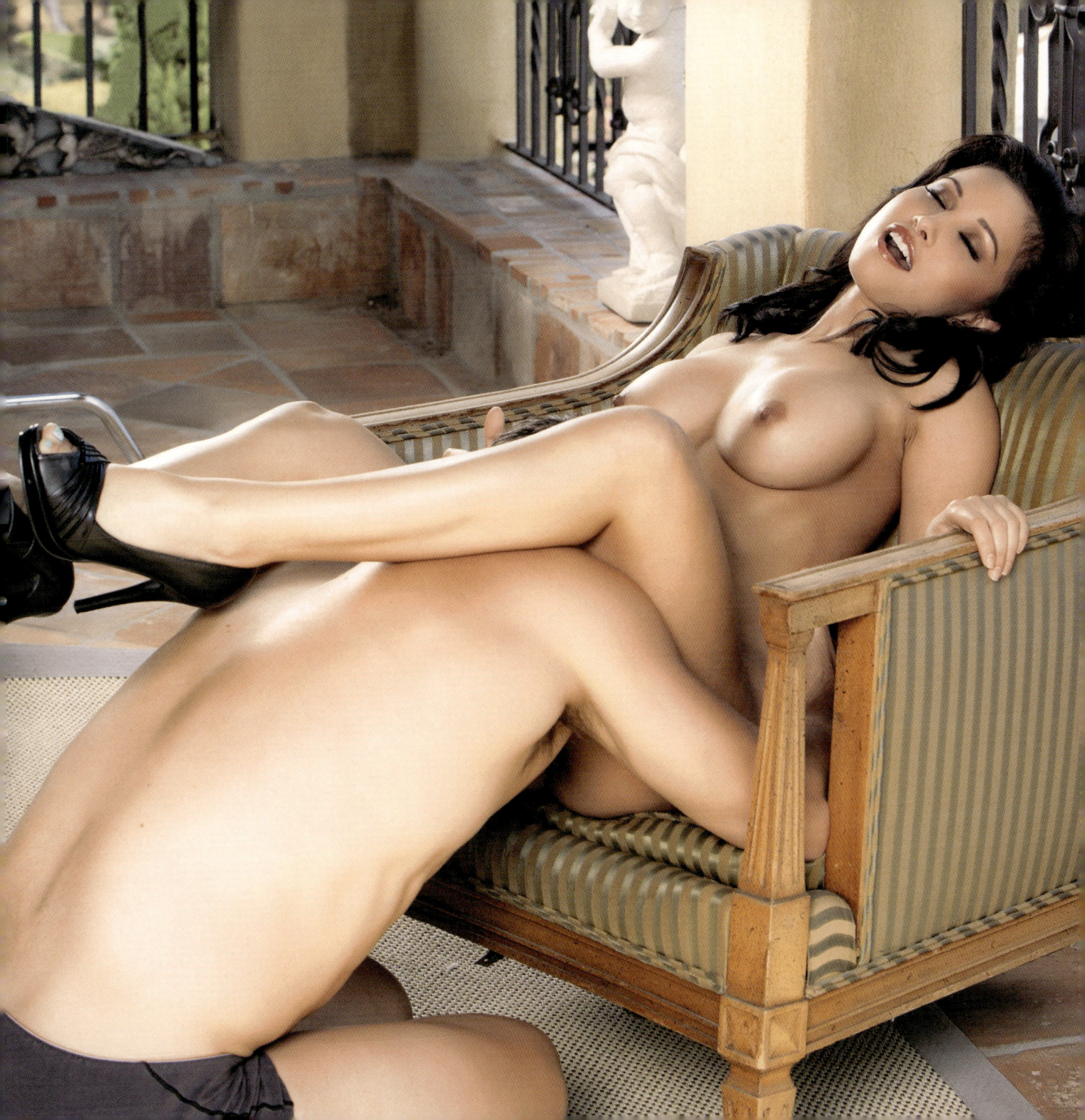

Jiggler. You might want to practice this inside her mouth first, to get warmed up. Jiggle your tongue side to side as fast as you can. Now apply this action to her labia, beginning at the bottom and gradually working your way up to the sensitive hood over her clitoris and then, finally, to the clitoris itself. (If direct clitoral contact is just too much for her, confine your jiggling to the prepuce—she'll still feel it through and through.) Slowly move your head up toward her abdomen and back down toward her buttocks, jiggling all the while, to stimulate the entire genital area. You are a human vibrator—and she'll love every minute of it.

Deep Thrust. Your tongue isn't your penis—but it can act like one. The sensation is different but equally wonderful. Thrust your tongue into her vagina, starting with just the tip and gradually increasing the pressure and depth. Alternate this with some tongue circles around the opening and some quick flicks over the hood of the clitoris. Heaven!

Hand to Mouth. There's no reason why you have to choose between tongue action and manual stimulation—try both at once. Use your hands to spread and stroke her labia while your tongue explores the inner reaches; insert a finger into her vagina while licking rings around it, or insert the tip of your thumb just a little way into her opening and press down while your tongue presses and laps upward against her clitoris. Working together, your hands and mouth can cause a sensation.

Penis Power

And while we're walking the line between foreplay and sex: Did you know that you could use your penis as an instrument of pleasure—without penetration? Use that magic wand of yours creatively and drive your lover wild.

Grasp your (by now erect) penis with one hand and wield it like a sword, starting at her belly button. Press in with the tip, gradually moving it down to her mound, jabbing and circling at your whim. Employ some gentle jabs to her engorged mound, then begin circling her vagina, using your powerful penis to toy with her labia, tease her clitoris, and even flirt with her anus. (You are probably lubricated by a bit of pre-come, but if not, feel free to apply some saliva or light lube.) Roll her over and slap her behind with it. Wag that member back and forth across her swollen lips until she begs for more.

Just for Women: Your Pleasure Guide to *Him*

Okay, ladies, it is your turn at bat. And since turnabout is fair play, here's your own anatomical guide to your lover, naming all of the key parts in question (see illustration):

That's the landscape, inside and out. Some of this information may seem like extra details, but be aware that some of what you do to stimulate his outer parts will exert pressure on what lies inside—so it's important to know where it all is and how it feels. (You might even want to share this diagram with your lover; many men don't understand their own bodies any more than you do.) Men carry more of their sex organs outside the body than women do, but that doesn't mean they are without mysteries.

Your man may or may not be circumcised, but that shouldn't affect your play down there too much. If he has his foreskin, your manipulation of his penis will involve the movement of that hood up and down; if he's without foreskin, your hands or mouth will be moving against the bare shaft. Either way, it'll feel fantastic to him. Most agree that a man's sexual responsiveness is neither hampered nor heightened by the presence of foreskin (and if it is a bit different, he'll have no basis for comparison in any case). So let's take the plunge:

Just Looking. Start out by looking at him rather than touching. Spread your lover's legs wide, kneel between them, and take a loving look at all his manly parts. He may be soft, semi-hard, or hard as a rock at this point, but your gaze alone will stimulate him—and you. Check out his penis, run your hand over his pubic hair, and softly fondle the globes of his testicles. If he's been circumcised, the head or glans of the penis is probably looking right back at you, the testicles already tensing up toward his body, the rush of blood flushing the entire area.

Jiffy Lube. Before you lay a hand on your man, dip into your favorite lube. Unlike you, your lover dispenses very little of his own lubrication—just a bit of what is known as pre-come—so his crankshaft and gears probably need a bit of oil to operate, just like a car does. Once your hands are slicked up (you'll probably be using both of them), start with the most obvious place: the shaft of his penis.

One-Ring Circus. First, make the "okay" sign—forming a ring with your thumb and forefinger—and surround the shaft with it at its base, near where it joins his balls. Now squeeze gently and run that ring up and down his penis. As you go over the "hump"

or corona that connects the head to the shaft, increase the pressure a little bit; this is a deliciously sensitive part, especially on the backside or frenulum area. (Ultimately, it is stimulation there that causes orgasms in most men, but let's not get ahead of ourselves.) Increase and decrease the pressure as you move up and down the shaft. Vary the speed, as well, but find a rhythm he enjoys.

Fiery Fists. Next, try this same movement using your entire hand, relubricating when necessary and paying close attention to your lover's responses. If your goal is to excite him without bringing him to orgasm (usually the case during foreplay, though not always), then be sure to hold back or change technique if you sense he's close to coming. Not sure? Murmur in his ear and ask for confirmation.

Rhythm Section. As you stroke his penis with your hand, find a nice rhythm and stick with it for awhile; switch hands intermittently or work with both hands in rapid succession. Try alternating only down strokes—but be careful with this one if you don't want him to come yet!

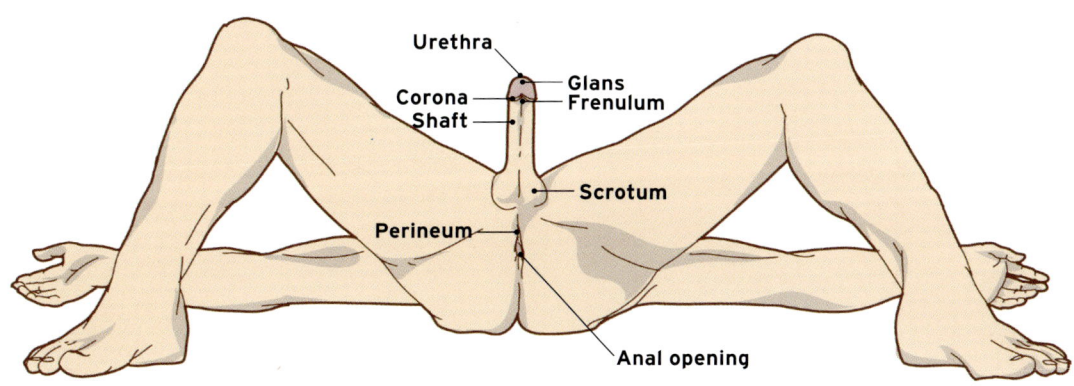

Do the Twist. Use a twisting movement with your hands as you move up and down, or add a "drumming" motion by varying the pressure exerted with each individual finger successively.

B-Side Bliss. Concentrate on the back of the penis to add variation, running one finger straight up and down, then in snaky curves. (Back there, less can be more—so be gentle unless he tells you otherwise.) Run your fingertip around and around the corona and head, pausing to pick up some of that juicy pre-come from the very tip for natural lubrication.

Twist-Off Cap. Pretend the glans is the top of a jar or bottle and (gently!) twist your hand as if you are twisting it off and on.

Have a Ball. Ready to give his shaft a break? Take some time to get to know his balls—they are delightfully sensitive as well. Cup each one in your hand, feeling its weight, shape, and orange-skin texture. The testicles have plenty of extra skin, just as the penis does, so they can expand and contract. Sometimes, they will feel loose and saggy, and other times round, taut, and closer to the body. They are often asymmetrical, too, with one larger than the other—but they are always responsive, so never leave them out of the game of foreplay. Note that the testicles can be ticklish! Stroke them, jiggle them, bounce them, and run your thumb around them where they join his body. Watch him for positive responses or murmur "How's that?" from time to time.

Pleasure Path. Explore his perineum, the area between the base of his penis and his anus. Start by moving your fingers up his perineum. This area can handle a fair amount of pressure, so bear down a little, using some extra lube to help you slide your fingers smoothly toward his anus. Move your fingers back and forth, enjoying its slickness.

The Male G-Spot. Here's one of the big differences between men and women: Men have a prostate gland, which is responsible for storing and secreting the fluid that carries the sperm. That may not sound very sexy, but in fact stimulating the prostate (along his perineum or through his anus) can be extremely enjoyable—and the area inside his body adjacent to the prostate gland is actually called the male G-spot. Light pressure and repetitive circling near the prostate gland can be a mind-blowing new sensation for him—and might just bring your man to orgasm before you can count to three. They don't call it "milking" the prostate for nothing. (And if milking the prostate to orgasm isn't the goal, then use restraint.) Some men can feel this magic spot through the perineum, so try to find it by applying pressure there first. But the anal method is surefire *fire*.

Anal Made Easy. Anal play offers a range of new sensations for foreplay. Start by making sure that everything is clean and well-lubricated, then run a finger around his anal opening, teasing it open.

Venturing Inside. When you feel he is ready, gently insert one slippery fingertip—just a little way at first. Keep your finger still for a few seconds until he relaxes and opens up; then twist your finger a bit, gauging his response. If he seems to enjoy this touch, deepen your penetration and increase your movement very slowly.

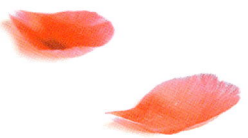

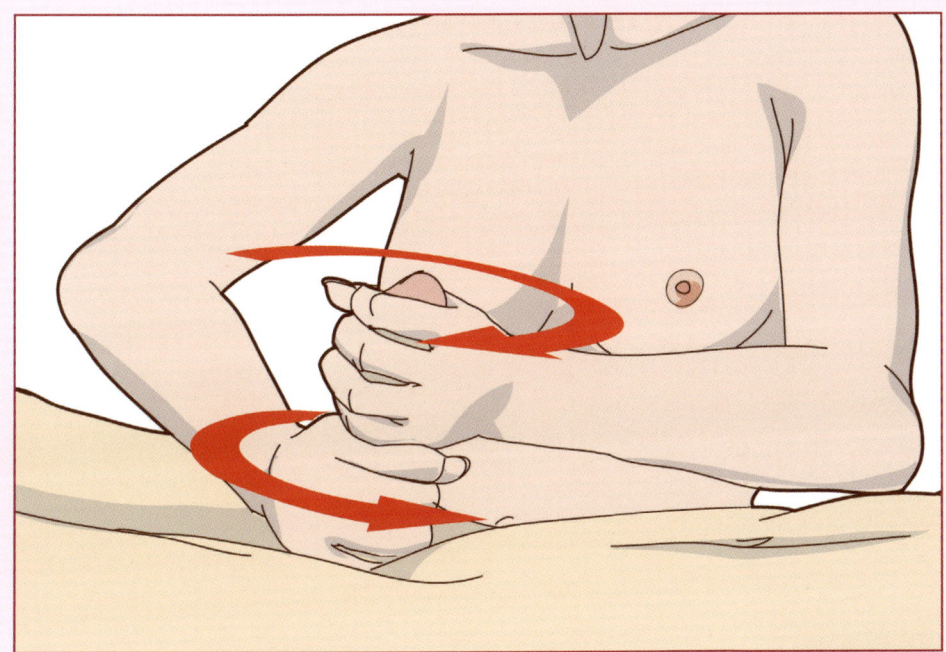

Do the Twist

Add a twisting motion to your stroke. This is certain to highten his arousal, but make sure you maintain adequate lubrication throughout.

Pleasure Path

Use your hand to explore his perineum, the area between the base of his penis and his anus.

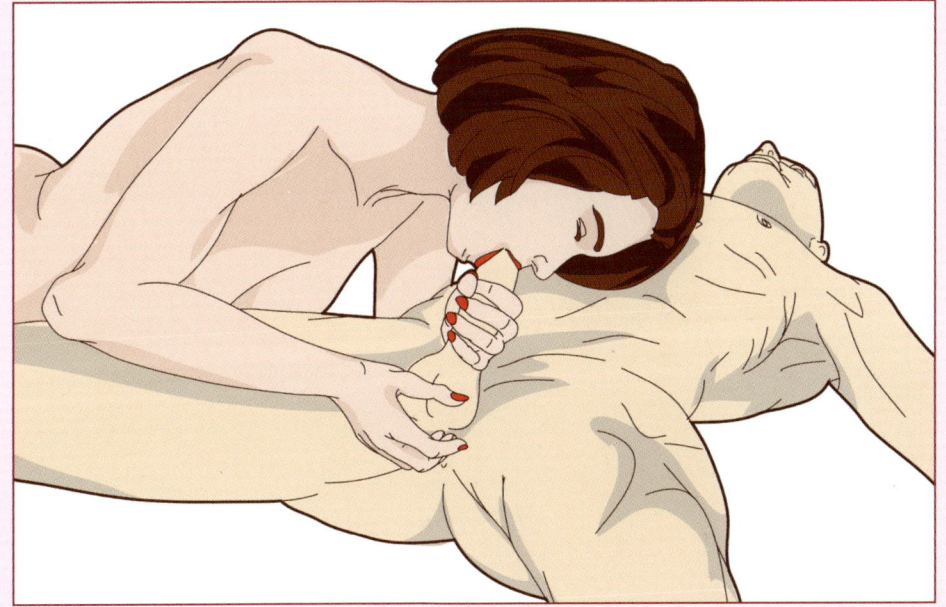

Intro to Oral: Ladies' Division

As I said in the men's section, though this isn't a book *about* oral sex, it seems wrong to leave the neighborhood without giving a taste of what's available. Here are a few basic oral techniques you can use when it's time to get this party started:

Keep the Tip. Grasp the shaft of his penis with one hand and run the tip of your tongue around its sensitive head. Circle it, flick it teasingly with your tongue, and dart the very tip of your tongue gently in and out of the urethral opening. Close your lips around the head of the penis and suck on it gently, then bob up and down on just the head, all the while using your tongue to circle the ever-so-sensitive corona.

Shaft Circle. Circle the base of his penis with your thumb and forefinger for stability, then circle the shaft with your tongue, moving up and down as you go round and round. As you reach the apex, slap it with the flat of your tongue, then return to circling.

Long and Luscious. Keeping your tongue as flat as you can, lap the backside of his shaft from base to tip. Start with a slow steady rhythm, then speed up, making your tongue into more of a point to increase pressure on the sensitive line up the center. Take breaks to explore his balls with your tongue, or alternate between this long, lapping motion and quick, all-over flicks.

Corn Cob. Want to try something different? Move your mouth or lips back and forth on his shaft as if you were sucking or nibbling a cob of corn. Every fourth or fifth journey, continue up and over to take the head of his penis in your mouth, then return to the corn cob movement. He's sure to writhe with delight.

Have a Ball. The testicles can seem particularly mysterious to women, since we have nothing like them—but they are extremely erogenous and can be downright sexy. Explore them with your hands first, feeling their weight and roundness. Stroke them lightly with your fingers, then let your mouth get in on the act, kissing, flicking, or poking them gently with your tongue, and finally lapping them vigorously. And don't play favorites: Go to work on both. You'll get plenty of positive feedback for this one.

Themes and Variations

Now that we've gone over the basics for each of you, here are some ideas you can both use. Think of these suggestions as inspiration for dreaming up your own stimulating fun—always keeping the safety and pleasure of your partner in mind:

Touch of Mink. In addition to your bare hands, there are lots of things you can use on your partner to vary sensations and produce a few chills. Try draping some silk panties or a scarf over your hand and using that on his or her nether parts. Ladies, wrap that silk scarf around his shaft and his balls; men, run the silk scarf teasingly over her clitoris. Ladies, if you have long hair, use it to stroke or even whip his penis and balls. Gentlemen, try running a string of beads between your lover's legs, allowing them to graze her engorged labia and clitoris. (Don't use real pearls, though—they might discolor.) Increase the friction as she desires.

Deep Breath. Use your breath as well as your hands: Blow, breathe, and exhale over your partner, and he or she will moan with delight.

Warm Feelings. Warm your hands with friction, or over a lit candle or radiator, before you touch any of your lover's sensitive areas. The extra warmth will add to the inner fire you are kindling and feel great on exposed skin.

Alternate Spot. The urethral opening, where your urine comes out, can be an erotic spot for some. Use a well-lubricated finger to experiment with some gentle circling, penetration, or massage.

Butt I Insist. Both of you: Don't skimp on your partner's buttocks. Massage, caress, fondle, slap, stroke, even bite the buttocks as part of genital play.

Spoonful. Remember that most things you can do face to face can also be accomplished in the spoon position—side by side, one of you behind the other, either lying down or sitting, and reaching around. This can be very unifying, making you feel wrapped up and melded into one person.

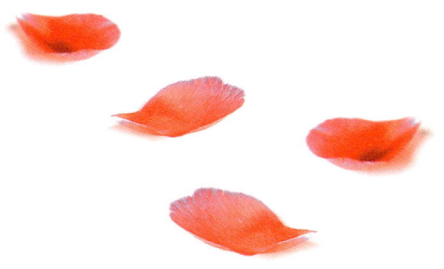

Alone Together: Enjoying Masturbation During Foreplay

Let's start with the facts: Self-pleasuring can be an empowering, deeply satisfying experience. It can teach you about your own responses and make you more receptive to pleasure and orgasm during sex (not, as that old myth would have it, *less* responsive).

I'm going to assume that both of you have masturbated regularly, and that you have found the methods of pleasuring yourself that you most enjoy. If that's not the case and you'd like an introductory course in self-satisfaction, there are any number of books that deal with the basics. (Check out *The Better Sex Guide to Extraordinary Lovemaking*, for one.) In any case, there's no harm in expanding your horizons, so don't hesitate to experiment with new positions and strokes, on your own or during foreplay.

If you are nervous about engaging in this intimate performance for your lover, practice in front of a mirror. This will surely make you more comfortable with the idea and will probably teach you a thing or two about your own anatomy and desires. Remember that self-love begins with self-knowledge, so admire the view.

Including masturbation in foreplay serves several purposes: It is a sexy, liberating performance for your partner; it will clue him or her in to the kinds of touch you like best; and of course it will take your arousal up a notch, since nobody knows your body and how to rev it up better than you do. This shouldn't surprise you: Studies have shown that people who masturbate regularly to orgasm have many more orgasms with their partners.

To get the show-and-tell session going, sit or lie back and start to fondle yourself in your favorite way while locking eyes with your lover. You might want to start with some clothes on—there's nothing sexier than stroking yourself through your silk panties and feeling them get slick with your juices. Reach inside your underwear, veiling your exact movements from your lover for a moment. Let your feelings show on your face: You are enjoying your own touch, so tell him so with your eyes, your tongue (lick those lips), your moans, and your sighs.

Now, get those panties off and get rid of the obstructed view. Ladies, if you are fingering or palming your labia and clitoris, show him how fast and in what specific way. If you like a finger or two inside you, make sure he can see exactly how you move it in, out, and roundabout. Gentlemen, how do you like your penis stroked? Instead of directing her, this is your chance to show her your favorite technique: Long strokes? Quick pumping?

Remember that masturbating for or with your lover is not quite the same as doing it alone. When we're on our own, we sometimes want to be efficient or goal-oriented about it, making ourselves come as quickly as we can. That's not usually the idea during foreplay. Go slowly, dramatically; have fun showing off your beautiful organs and the way they respond to stimulation. Maybe you want to come for your lover—or maybe you want to hold back until she is touching you, tasting you, or enveloping you.

You can take turns masturbating for each other or do it at the same time. (If one of you starts, chances are the other will want to get in on the act.) And don't forget to get your whole body involved. Stroke your breasts, squeeze your nipples, run your free hand over your body in ways you enjoy, paying particular attention to your favorite sensual spots. Your lover will surely be taking note of all the stunning details.

As for positions, that is entirely your call (though, ladies, if your position of choice when alone is flat on your stomach or in "doggie" position, with your hand under your body, you might want to try something more showy for this purpose). Sitting, reclining, standing, lying on your back with your knees pulled up—try whatever makes you comfortable and makes for a good show.

Do you like to use a dildo, vibrator, or other sex toy while you masturbate? Feel free to break it out when your lover is present, too. It could lead you down a whole new avenue together. (For more on sex toys, see chapter 6.)

Fantasy and masturbation go together—and that doesn't change when you are in the same room with your lover. Go ahead and let your imagination roam free—you can fantasize about each other and the wild sex that's soon to come, or about anyone and any setting you choose. Remember that the mind is the most erogenous zone of all, and there's never any need to hold back on what goes on in there.

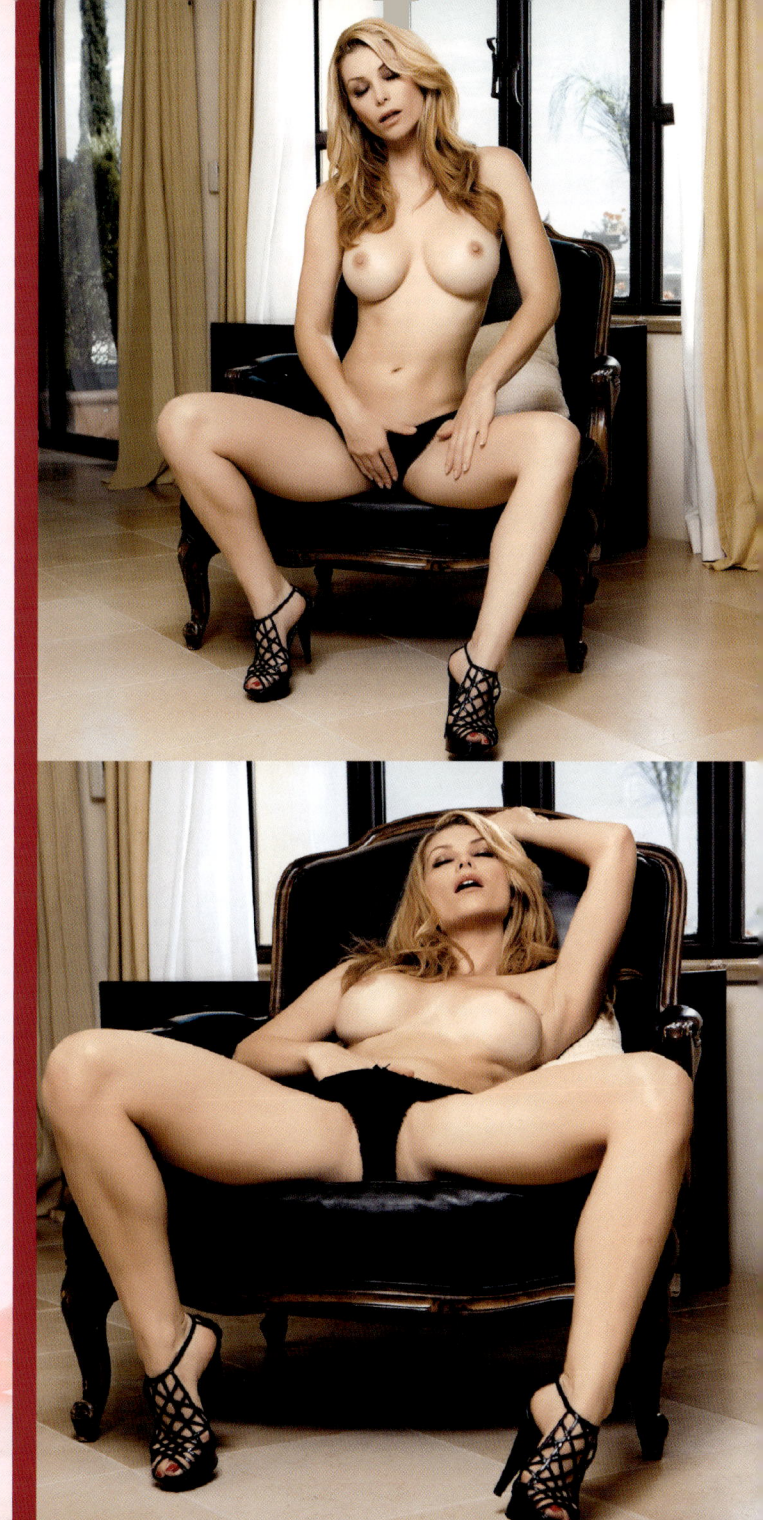

Rocking Role-Play

Now that you've expanded your repertoire of touch techniques and augmented your ideas about when, where, and how to engage in fabulous foreplay, it's time to step out and enjoy the supersexy world of role-play.

Pretending to be someone else for a little while can be extremely liberating. Think about it: That character you're playing might be willing to do all kinds of things you wouldn't! Taking on a new role can help you let your guard down for a little while, explore more adventurous ways of thinking and behaving—and give your mate an opportunity to get it on with a "stranger"!

Role-play is a great way to spice up a relationship, particularly a long-term one, and keep things from getting too predictable. Talk over the idea as a couple and, if you are both comfortable with it, start thinking of some scenarios you'd both enjoy.

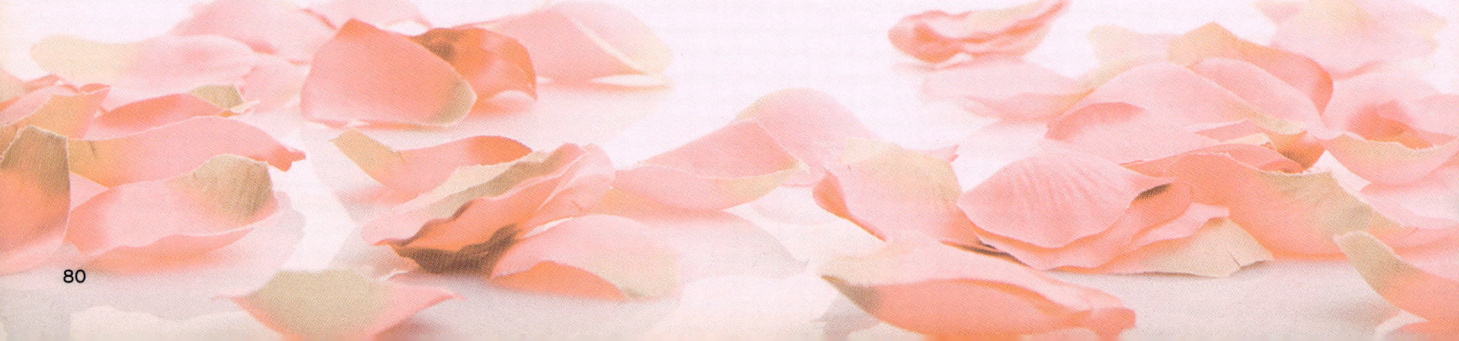

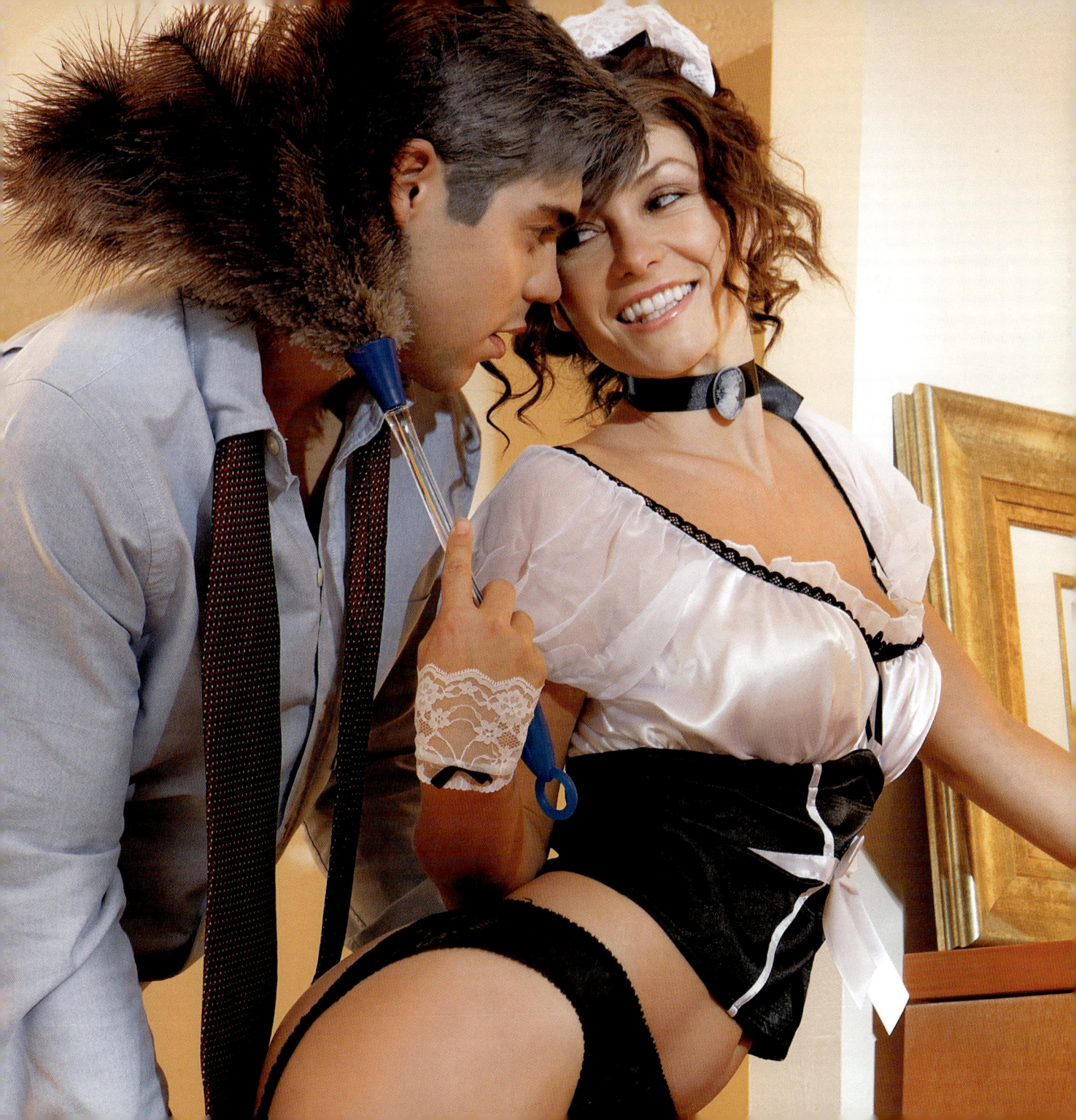

Turnabout Is Fair Play

One way to ease into role-playing is to start by simply switching roles. You become him and he becomes you. Guys, if you think you'll feel strange pretending to be your lady love (with or without the clothes, shoes, and makeup), you might surprise yourself. Especially when she swaggers into the room as *you* and starts the action by manhandling you in all of the ways she herself loves. "Hey, beautiful, come over here and give your husband a kiss" might start the ball rolling, and you'll find yourself being tossed onto the bed and groped by your "manly" mate. Ladies, play the role to the hilt, including a rolled sock under your fly that you can press into him suggestively as you pin his hands over his head and use his favorite moves to seduce him.

Guys, dressing up in things from your lady's closet can be fun. The feel of her silk panties or nightgown against your skin and the whiff of her scent will turn you on. When she enters the room, get down on your pretty knees and offer to give her the best blow job she's ever had—and then do it, just as she would.

This particular game doesn't have to be about dressing in drag—it can just be a simple exercise in empathy, made hot and steamy by enacting those fantasies of what you'd do if *you were him* or if *you were her*. Just as in the masturbation game in the last chapter, this is an opportunity to learn more about what turns your lover on—this time by seeing how he or she behaves when the tables are turned.

Fantasy Threesome

You may not be ready for a real threesome, but you can pretend, can't you? Played to the hilt, this scenario can be hot and satisfying for both of you.

First, decide who is taking the lead. (In this example, ladies, we'll put you in charge.) Lead your man into the bedroom and make sure he's comfortable. This isn't a dress-up affair—I suggest few or no clothes. Next, lower the lights and slip a blindfold on him, telling him that you don't want to ruin the surprise. Tell him that you've invited another woman to join the two of you for a sexy romp—and she's waiting in the hallway. Before you "let her in," describe her, detailing her many lovely features—dark eyes, long blonde hair, shapely breasts and behind, skin-tight skirt, silk stockings—whatever you think will turn him on most. She can be a beautiful stranger, or she might even be someone you think he fantasizes about, such as a movie star or the cocktail waitress at your local bar. Be sure to call her by her name. Then open the door and invite her in, introduce her to your lover, and close the door behind her.

Since your man can't see, you'll have to describe everything, even as you play the roles of both women. "Angelina looks so gorgeous—she's wearing skin-tight jeans, black leather high-heeled boots, and a see-through silk blouse. I'm unbuttoning the blouse for her now, and mmm, I can't resist reaching in to feel her round, lovely breast . . ." Describe how your new friend undresses then approaches him. Meanwhile, of course, you perform all the actions yourself.

Really make him believe he is being attended to by his sexy fantasy lover while you watch—and take the opportunity to touch him and pleasure him in new ways. Don't use the moves he's accustomed to from you, but really try to make him believe he's being serviced by a luscious wench he's never met. If you usually shy away from licking his balls and asshole, do it with relish now. If you rarely make sounds as you pleasure him, moan and sigh. Dangle your breasts in front of his waiting lips and make him suck your nipples. Really *be* someone else, and sense the freedom and power that comes from role-playing.

Tell him it is his moment to just enjoy himself and not worry about giving pleasure in return. Tell him how much you are enjoying the show. "Watching Angelina stroke your cock is getting me so wet, I have to reach down and wipe the liquid from my dripping pussy. Would you like a taste?" At the same time, play the role of the serving girl to the max: Stroke his cock with one hand while you finger his anus with the other; squeeze his ass cheeks and make him thrust his cock deep into your mouth, then hold on with your lips as you slide it out. Do as many different things with your hands and mouth as you can manage to really give him a sense that there are two ladies present.

Then, if you think he'll like it (and what man doesn't?), take it up a notch by telling him that you've caught the eye of your new lady friend and it's your turn for action. Describe for him all the things the two of you ladies are doing to each other. Are you kissing passionately? Stroking each other's breasts and buttocks? Tasting each other's delicious bodies? As you talk about it, feel free to pleasure yourself so all of those delighted moans and sighs will be real. And encourage him to touch himself, as well. Pretty soon, you'll both be in ecstasy, lost in the fantasy of your perfect threesome.

It takes a little creativity, but conjuring up that third person for your lover's pleasure can be a rewarding fantasy for both of you. Soon, you'll be asking her to leave, so to speak, and tearing off his blindfold. You'll be going at it with newfound gusto.

Next time around, the blindfold will be on *you*, and it will be your man's turn to invite a secret guest in to share the fun—male or female!

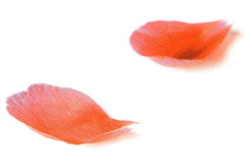

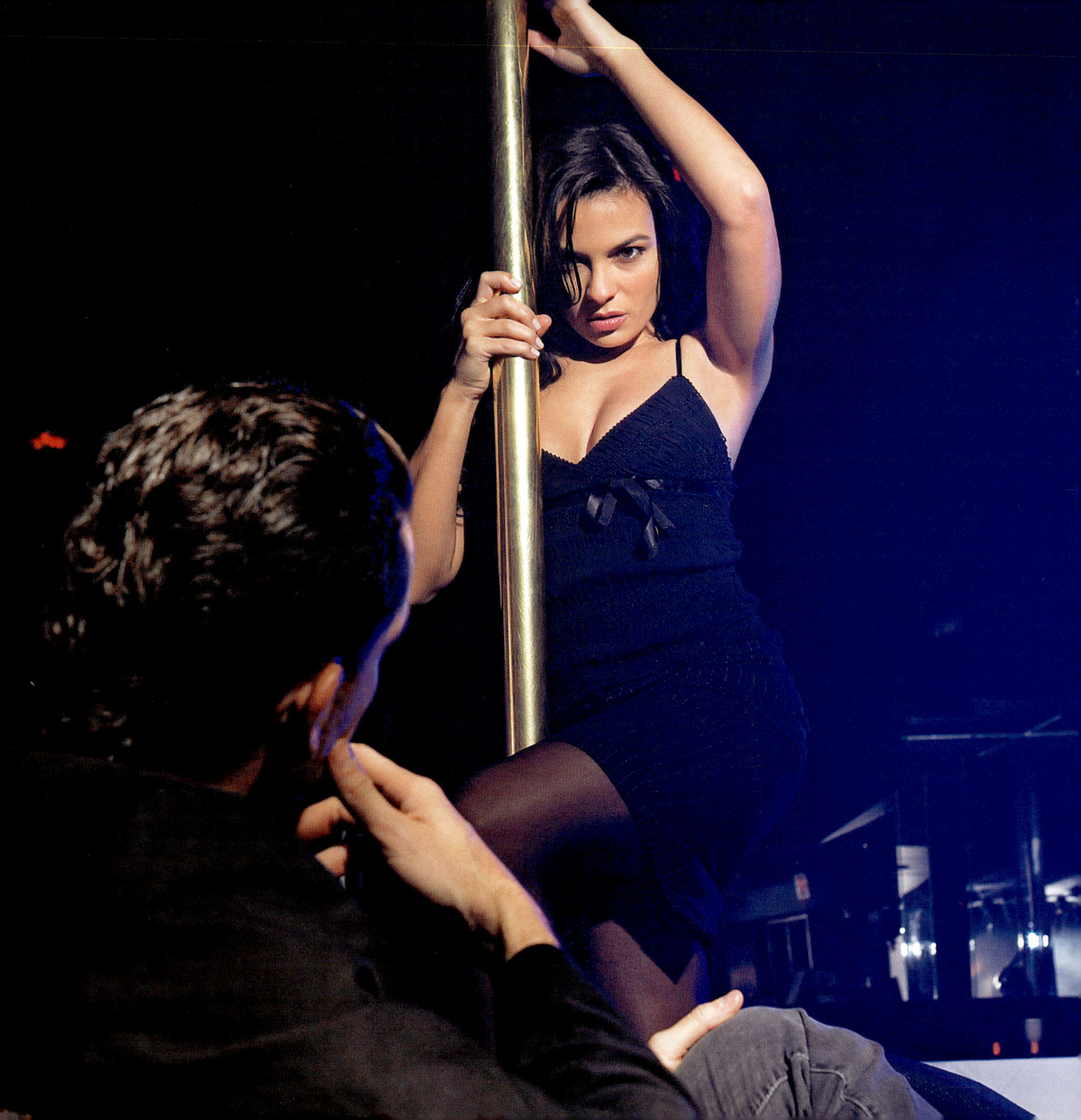

Lights, Camera, Action

Guys, we'll give you a turn with this one (though either of you can take the lead in most of these scenarios). The setup here is that you are making a porn film or taking pornographic photos. You are the director and your lover is the beautiful star, a veteran porn queen who knows all the moves and loves to perform for the camera.

First, arrange the bedroom as your set, complete with bright lights focused on the bed. Don't forget the luxurious props, such as a fur throw, silk sheets, and lots of fluffy pillows. Alternatively, set your scene on a couch or fur rug in front of a roaring fire.

If you are taking still shots, tell her they are for a high-class porn magazine. Have her leave some clothes on at first and lie back with her legs spread, facing you. Ask her to start by pulling her panties aside to show the camera what is underneath. Get her on her knees, doggy-style, so she can show off her luscious breasts for the camera. Break out some props—handcuffs, a dildo, or a vibrator—and position her in various poses, using the devices on herself. Make sure her face reflects her emotions, too, so she acts the role to the hilt.

For movies, you can use a real camera to film the action if you want to, or you can fake it—but take your role as a director seriously and make it clear to your lover that she must act every inch the porn star or she'll be fired. Dress for your part, too—the all-business director. And do your homework—if you are taking real footage, study some porn films and magazines for ideas about sets, props, and provocative positions.

Your film star should be in a bathrobe with nothing underneath, or with her sexiest set of undies, stockings, high heels—whatever getup feels most authentic for both of you. Make sure she knows who is boss. Tell her that, as director, you are totally in charge and she must do whatever you desire. Run her through some moves to get her warmed up: Have her fondle her breasts and twist her nipples, flutter her clitoris, and insert several fingers into her vagina to get herself wet and ready. Now tell her to lie cheek-down with her ass high in the air, pointed toward the camera, and turn her face toward you so she's looking into the camera. Since this is a film, you need action—so give her her favorite dildo and instruct her to use it on herself and be enthusiastic about it.

Once you've put her through some moves, describe a scenario for her. Perhaps she is a young newlywed, waiting impatiently for her husband to come home so she can surprise him at the door. Or she is a prostitute waiting for her customer to arrive.

Start rolling by yelling "Action," and then continue to direct her through the scene. Perhaps her husband calls on the phone—he's going to be late! Hmm, what can a sex-crazed young girl do? She'll just have to start without him. Direct your porn star to pleasure herself for the camera, and tell her not to hold back on her reactions. Have her start with her fingers, trying out all of her favorite masturbation techniques and positions. You might want to have her move on to a dildo, vibrator, or other sex toy—after all, you're the director, and what you say goes.

You can end the scene at any point and get her onto the "casting couch"—or you can take on the role of the "husband" yourself and finish out the scene as two actors performing for the camera. You'd be surprised how ingenious you two can be when you imagine those cameras rolling!

Though you are playing roles, the camera can be real. As director, you can choose to really film your star using your own digital camera—but if you do, be careful to keep the results someplace secure and private. You wouldn't want your children or parents to come across the footage when looking for vacation pictures! But by all means enjoy the show whenever the fancy strikes you. Next time, men, it'll be your turn under the lights.

An Apple for the Teacher

The teacher-student scenario is a classic with many variations. Either one of you can play the teacher, and you can express whatever personality you choose in the role—from mousy to domineering. Likewise, your student can be obedient and shy, rebellious and bold, or anything in between. This is a really good scenario to get the action going, bringing back all of those feelings you experienced as sexy young things in homeroom.

In this example, let's put the lady at the front of the classroom. You are a high-school teacher—a hot one that your hormone-rich boy students dream about—so dress the part: tight blouse with select buttons open, slim skirt, stockings, and heels. Your student is a sweet, smart boy who sits in the front row during English class; his long eyelashes and soulful eyes have captivated you since the first day of school—but of course you would never do anything about those naughty feelings. Or would you?

This scene is most easily set in your living room. You probably don't have a blackboard—you can mime that part—but feel free to find something you can use as a pointer. (It might come in handy later, if you need to deliver a playful little spanking.) Your "student" should be dressed in a simple shirt and jeans or khakis and sneakers. Add a pair of glasses if that turns you on. Begin by giving your student a bit of a scolding. "This is the second time this week you've come in without your assignment completed," you say, or something to that effect. "I'm afraid I'm going to have to keep you after class so we can get to the bottom of it."

"Yes, ma'am," replies your student, and waits obediently for the rest of the class to leave.

Now heat things up. Start by asking him to erase the chalkboard for you, and admire his tight behind as he does it. (He's the captain of the swim team, after all.) "You are very fit, young man . . . I must confess you are starting to turn me on." Come up behind him, touch his shoulder, graze your hand over his ass. As he turns around to face you, his adolescent feelings overwhelm him. He grabs your shoulders, pulls you in for a kiss, and soon he is pinning you against the wall, tearing open your blouse, plunging his hands inside your bra, then his mouth. "Now let's see how you can bring up your grade," you tell him. "Start by unzipping those pants and letting me see what you've got." From there, I'm sure you can use your imagination, playing out that teacher-student role for all it's worth.

Alternatively, maybe things start more slowly. He confesses to you that he can't concentrate in class because he has a crush on you. "Is that an erection?" you ask him, grazing your hand across the growing bulge beneath his beltline. Drop to your knees and start polishing that apple he's brought just for you, right through his blue jeans. "Yes, ma'am . . . um, I'm sorry. I just get so excited when you wear that tight skirt. I really need to open my zipper a little bit—is that okay?" Tell him you'll be happy to do the honors—if he promises never to tell the other students—and then release his cock so you can take it in your hands, your mouth, and whatever strikes your fancy.

Whatever turn your scene takes, stay in character throughout. You are a teacher with a dirty mind and a stud or a student; he's young and awkward but a quick study, determined to learn all he can from his favorite teacher. You're having a furtive grope in the classroom, worried that at any moment the bell will ring and others will come in and discover your naughtiness. Enjoy! And when school's out, you'll be ready to do what you never learned in the classroom.

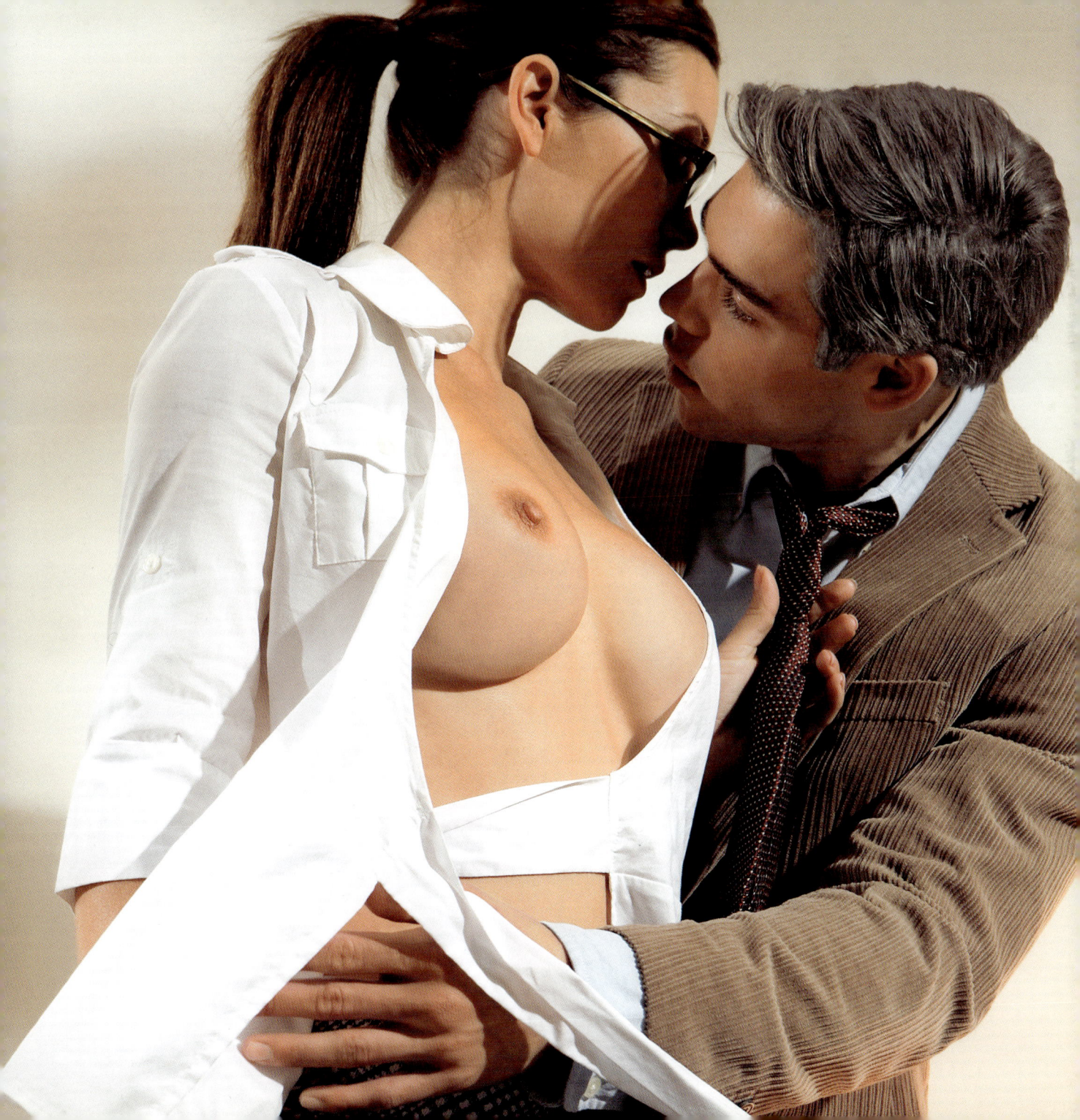

The Doctor Is *In*

Maybe you played a doctor game or two as kids—but now it's time to take that game to its adult limits.

Start by turning your bedroom into an examining room, taking all of the blankets off the bed and turning the bedside light up bright. Dress appropriately as male doctor and female patient, and proceed to your appointment. You are a shy, beautiful patient and your lover is a kind but firm physician. Go through the preliminaries of talking about your "condition," undressing (in private, of course—your closet or hallway can be a changing room), and putting on a gown. (You can use a nightgown for the purpose.)

"Oh, doctor, thanks for seeing me on such short notice. I can't imagine what could possibly be wrong, but I feel so strange . . . down there." And with that, you are off on a great fantasy where you ask the strong, handsome doctor to help you cure your "woman problem"—and he is more than happy to help you out. When you explain that you've been alone and without sex for awhile, he surmises correctly that your discomfort isn't life-threatening and can be easily alleviated. "What you need," says the wise doctor, "is some stimulation and some release." Using his gloved finger, he proceeds to attack your "problem," then moves on to several fingers and even some "instruments" you've gathered for the purpose. It's easy to see how this session can turn into some all-out fun, with great clinical results for both of you!

Visiting Nurse

Here's a variation on the doctor fantasy. This scenario might come in handy on a quiet afternoon. Tell your man you're going out for a bit, then dress up as a sexy, naughty nurse. White stockings and a red push-up bra and garters can complete the look. Add a toy doctor kit so you can bring along some useful props, including rubber gloves, lubricant, or a vibrator.

Ring the doorbell, and when your lover answers the door, announce that you're the visiting nurse come to follow up on his problem: low libido. Have him lie on the bed while you check him out. Undress him slowly and examine every inch of him, avoiding the genitals until he's squirming, all the while flashing him a peek of your lingerie or red bra. Then manhandle him until he's hot and ready.

The Cat Burglar Strikes Again

Who's that sneaking in through the window? Could it be . . . a cat burglar?

Switch up this classic fantasy by reversing the usual genders: Make it a lady burglar surprising an innocent, sleeping male victim. Dress in your tightest black jeans or leggings, a provocative black sweater, and a black eye mask. (You probably have one of those sleep masks from the last overseas flight you took, and you can cut eyeholes out of that, but if not, check out a costume shop, where you can find lots of great props and costume pieces for these scenarios and inspiration for others.)

Gentlemen, your role in this one is to climb under the covers (you sleep naked, right?) and go to sleep—or pretend to, anyway. In through the window or bedroom door creeps the most beautiful cat burglar ever, looking for goodies in the dresser drawers and nightstand. Despite her attempts to be quiet, you wake up and surprise her by throwing on the lights. Then there are a couple of ways you can go, depending on what turns you on. Perhaps you overpower her, tie her up, and toy with her until she stops struggling and begs for more. Or maybe she pulls out a (toy) gun and holds you at gunpoint, forcing you to do her bidding. In the battle of the burglar versus the victim, it is less important which of you has the ultimate upper hand than that you both have a ball while playing out your roles as bold aggressor and frightened captive.

Wherever you go with this fantasy of dominance and submission, it is bound to be a memorable and satisfying evening where both of you stretch the boundaries of your usual behavior. Sometimes crime *does* pay!

Special Delivery

Ding-dong. "Special delivery for *you!*"

When your man dresses up in tight shorts and a delivery cap, be sure to come to the door ready to receive the goods! This scenario has been a staple of porn films and salty stories since the invention of the truck—and for good reason. The idea of being ravished in the middle of the day by a deliveryman (or plumber, carpenter, mailman—whatever) is a potent fantasy shared by many women. Now is your chance to act it out and release your inner slutty housewife in the process.

When that handsome delivery guy comes to the door, the polite thing to do is invite him in, offer him a cold drink, and tell him you'll be right back because you want to get out of your sweaty workout gear and into something more comfortable. Leave him alone for a few minutes to think about how you must look as you strip off your sweats, and then reappear in your sexiest little sundress or short shorts. Sit *very* close to him on the couch and ask him about his day. Is it very hard heaving all of those boxes around? Would he like a shoulder massage to ease his tired muscles?

Start to work him over with a great back rub and see what develops. Suggest he take his shirt off—it's such a warm day, after all. Both of you should feel free to improvise within your roles and follow the scene wherever it leads. To the floor, couch, or kitchen table, I'm guessing! Don't forget to give him a nice tip for good service when you're all done.

Satisfaction Guaranteed

Guys, for this one you are going to dress up as a door-to-door salesman of sex toys! Pack up a "bag of tricks" ahead of time, with every sex toy you have—and maybe a few new ones purchased just for this game—and then surprise your lover when she thinks you're off at work or busy doing something else.

Ring the doorbell. When she answers, explain that you have some very exciting products to show her. Take out the toys one by one, explaining in detail what each one is for and how it can increase her pleasure.

Would she like a demonstration? No problem, but she must first strip naked. What's more, you're in charge—so once the demonstration begins, she must follow all your commands. If you want, pull out some silk ties or handcuffs and bind her arms or legs to a chair leg or bedpost to make sure she knows you mean business! Then run through your product line, taking your time to show her just how effective the devices are for stimulation, teasing, and perhaps even orgasm!

Sky's the Limit

Those are just a few classic role-playing scenes to get you started. With a little thought, you can come up with lots of your own—from the domineering chef and the sassy waitress to the traffic cop and the speeder. Each one takes a little bit of preparation to set the scene and get into character, but there's never a need for anything too elaborate or expensive: Your dirty minds are the best props you have, along with a sense of anything-goes fun. The freedom you'll feel from playing a role just might be addicting, but this kind of foreplay is *not* hazardous to your health. Enjoy it to the fullest.

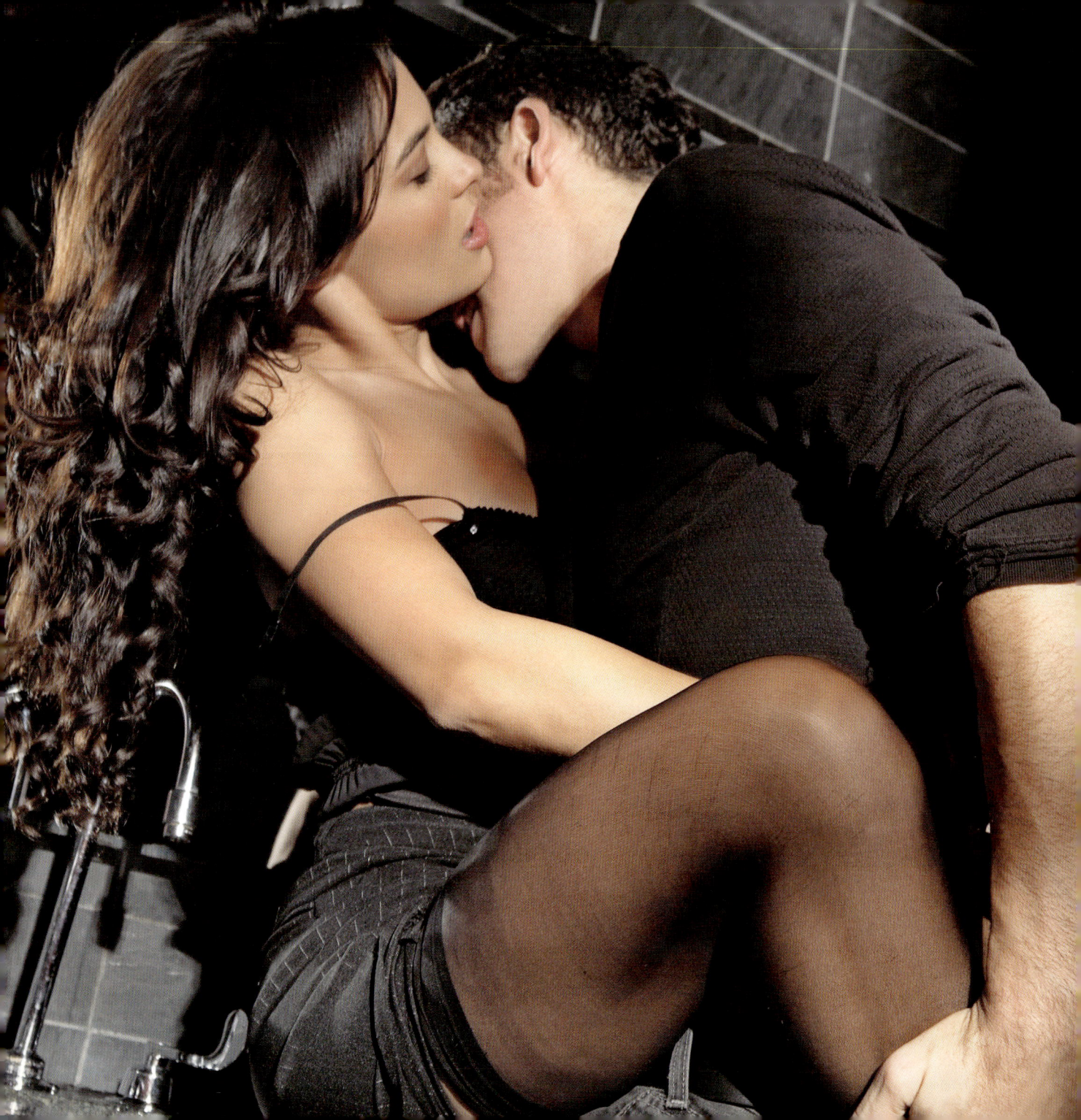

A Guy's Top Ten Fantasies—and How You Can Help Fulfill His Wildest Dreams

Being with His Favorite Movie Actress, Rock Star, or Other Celebrity. Find out who he admires, watch her in a movie or two, then dress and act like her for a night.

Having Two or More Women Catering to Him Simultaneously. Play the game described earlier, where you pretend to invite another woman to join you—or consider inviting a real-live woman along for foreplay!

Watching You with Another Woman (or Watching Two Women Together). If you have a friend you'd both feel comfortable inviting along, you have a chance to fulfill a fantasy he might never have thought he would have a chance to try.

Watching You with Another Man. Surprisingly, lots of guys like this one. If you aren't game to invite a third party along during foreplay, try blindfolding him and then describe what another man (George Clooney?) is doing to you.

Being Dominated—Even Tied Up, Blindfolded, Anally Violated, or Otherwise Dominated—by a Woman. Mistress fantasies are classic. Tailor any of the scenarios in this chapter so that you are the dominant one, or play a lady soldier, cop, CEO, or other boss figure.

Going Down a Line of Sexually Ravenous Women and Trying to Satisfy Them All. This one will take some doing, but you can always have a variety of outfits on tap, so he can have his way with a series of your alter egos.

Hiding Behind a Screen with Only His Lower Half Exposed, Being Serviced by One or More Women Who He Can't See and Who Can't See Him. You can act this one out by blindfolding him and playing a succession of different roles, each woman servicing him in a different way. Use different accents and a variety of his favorite techniques, from gentle to rough and tumble.

Having a Quickie in the Bathroom with a Stranger at a Bar, Movie Theater, or Other Public Place. Sex in public can be delicious fun for both of you—and you can always play the stranger. See Chapter 8 for all the ideas you will need to pull off a public encounter.

Having a Forbidden Affair with an Office Colleague, Boss, Underling, Kid's Teacher, Babysitter, or Other Associate. Again, play the role of that forbidden partner, whether it is a babysitter or a nun.

Sleeping with a Prostitute. There are lots of phone lines he can call for some naughty phone sex with a stranger. Pretend to be the person on the other end of the line, or if you really want to step it up, let him experience real phone sex. Give it your blessing, but tell him you want to listen in on the other extension. You might pick up some pointers from a pro!

A Gal's Top Ten Fantasies—and How You Can Help Fulfill Her Wildest Dreams

Having Sex with a Woman—or Several. Give her the go-ahead on this one, as long as you can be there to watch. If there's no other woman in the wings, blindfold her and play the role of a woman, ready to service her every need and desire.

Being with Her Favorite Movie Star, Politician, or Other Celebrity. The blindfold idea works for this one, as well. Now all you have to do is be Brad Pitt for a night!

Seducing (and Being Worshipped and Appreciated by) a Much Younger Man. Use that blindfold on her again and get ready to worship at the altar of pleasure.

Completely Dominating. Just say yes! Tell her that for a whole night, you will do whatever she asks—and promptly—from washing the dishes to giving her as many orgasms as she can handle, in whatever way she'd like them.

Seducing a Teacher, Doctor, Boss, or Other Forbidden Authority Figure. These are all roles you can play. Be extra convincing by using costumes, props, a different voice or accent—really be somebody else.

Having Dirty Sex with an Employee or Serviceman—Plumber, Gardener, Deliveryman, Pool Cleaner, and so on. Use costumes here, or just blindfold her and talk her through the fantasy.

Being Dominated, Tied Up, Blindfolded, or Otherwise Forced into Submission. Tie her up, handcuff her, spank her, give her orders. With you in charge, she can let go completely.

Being Taken Against Her Will. Yes, rape fantasies are okay. Tie her up, handcuff her, and take charge!

Selling Herself for Money. This scene will be fun for both of you, and it's best played out outside the house. Go to a bar and let her solicit you. Settle on a price and conditions, and then seal the deal.

Having Sex in Front of a Window, in a Public Place, or in Front of an Audience. Again, this one is easily fulfilled, either at home or, if you'd rather not involve the neighbors, at a local hotel.

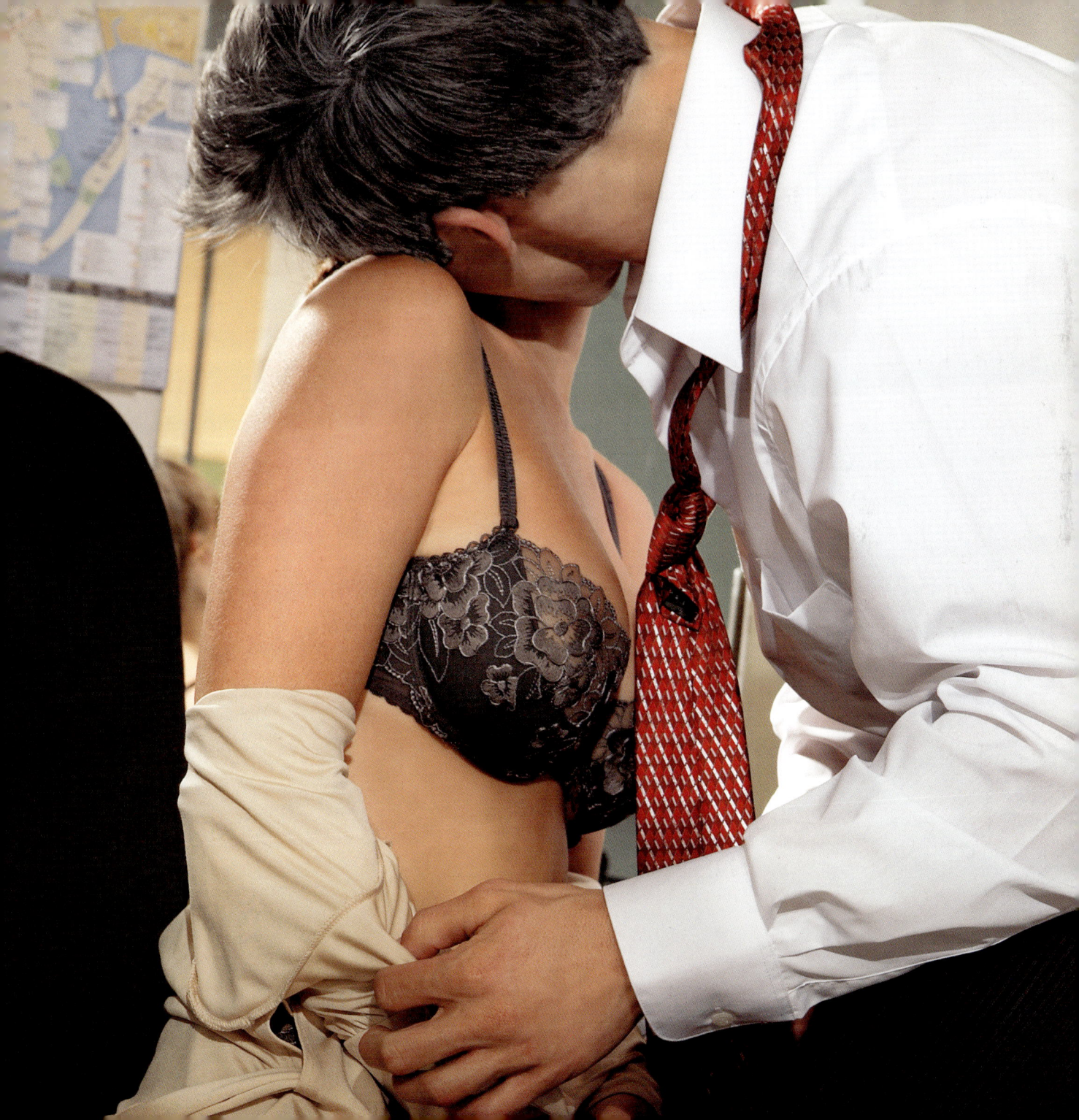

Tools, Toys, and Extra Credit

It's sometimes difficult to figure out the boundary between foreplay and sex (what a delightful boundary to breach!), but even in a book devoted to the preliminaries, it makes sense to touch on some of the more adventurous ways to get the party going full swing. After a few great experiences, just the sight of your own secret bag of tricks containing your favorite toys will be a turn-on for both of you.

We've already talked about role-playing, but there are lots of ways to take the games even further. And if you or your partner has always been a bit hesitant about shopping for or using toys and gear, or engaging in edgy activities, rest assured: This kind of equipment is safe and fun to shop for and use, and as long as your lines of communication are open and your mutual trust is secure, you can push the envelope with abandon. In fact, with the rise of e-commerce, you don't even have to leave the house to buy erotica or sex toys—unless you want to. (The shopping spree alone can be foreplay. Think about taking your lady-love shopping for some supersexy lingerie—and making her model the pieces you pick out.) But we're getting ahead of ourselves . . .

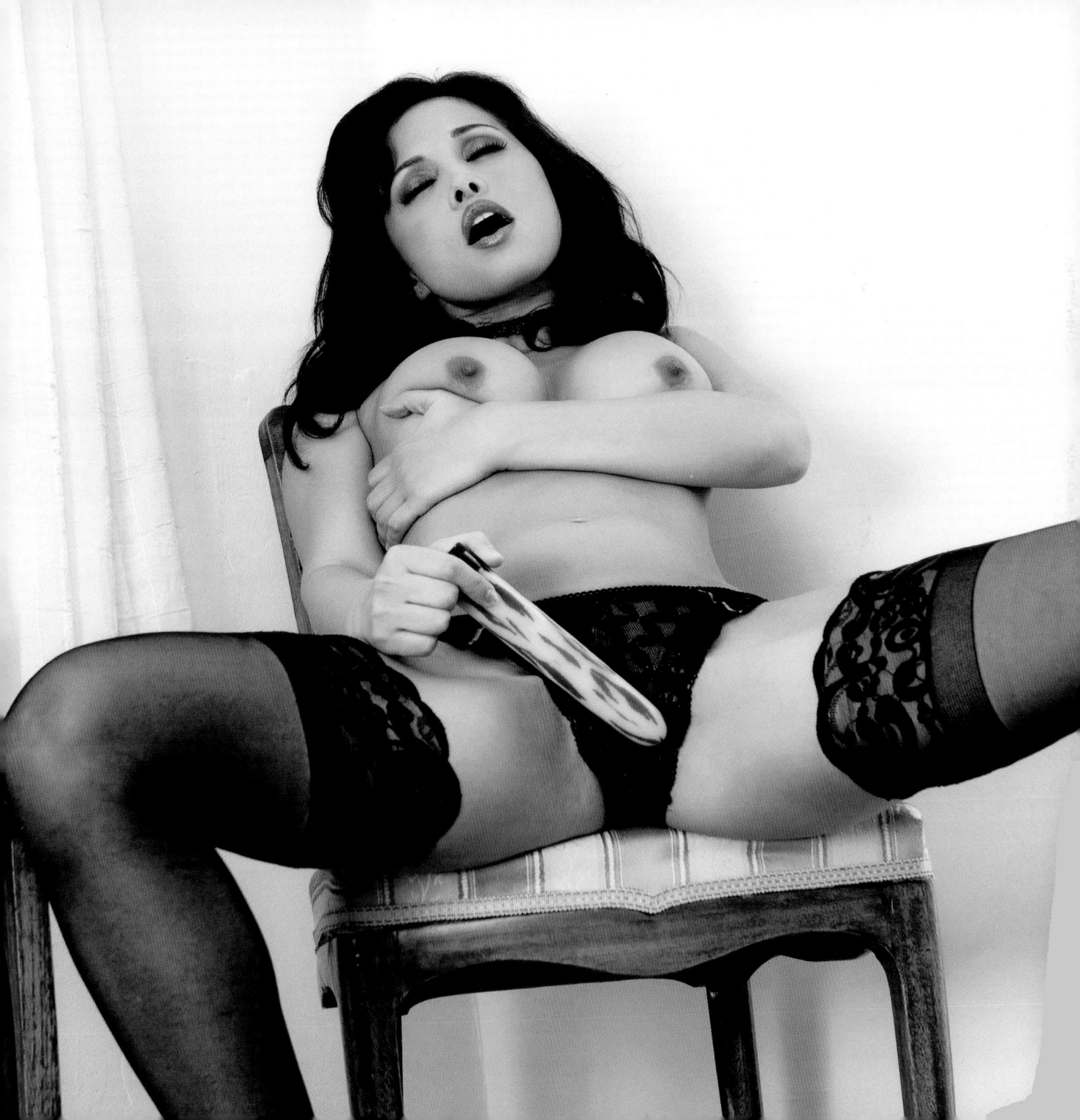

Getting Started—Talk It Over

One of the most common questions posed to sex columnists and therapists goes something like this: "I am interested in [bondage, sex toys, role-playing, S&M, whatever] but my [husband, wife, lover] has never indicated that [he, she] shares this interest. How do I get [him, her] to try this?"

Simple answer: It starts with a conversation. Choose a relaxed and neutral time to talk about sex—never when your lover is running out the door, and never ever during the heat of passion. Breakfast can be a nice time to broach the subject; cocktail hour is even better. Keep your tone and your words positive. Rather than saying, "How come you never want to try that strap-on I bought?" say, "Honey, you'd look so hot in that crazy strap-on! Maybe we should give it a whirl tonight." If you feel it will be helpful, rehearse what you want to say beforehand so it comes out in a loving way and not a critical one.

Be sure to listen as well as talk. Ask questions and make statements. It's likely that if you are heartfelt and honest, and bring things up in the spirit of mutual pleasure and satisfaction, your lover will be persuaded that trying something new or different could be fun. Make it clear that you are open to trying what he or she is interested in, too. And always, always stress the fact that you will never force your mate to do anything he or she is uncomfortable with. "Just say 'No' and it's game over." That should be a steadfast rule for both of you.

A great way to keep things safe when you are playing on the edge is to establish a safe word, something that either of you can say during the action that means "Stop right now—no kidding." You should choose something easy to remember, that wouldn't normally come up in the course of your sex play. Maybe "scrambled eggs," "shoe polish," or "lamppost." Then, in the course of the action, if you feel uncomfortable, unhappy, or in pain, just utter the magic word or words and your partner will back off immediately so you can regroup. Sex should never be scary or unpleasant.

Once you've talked everything over, agreed on some new activity (or outfit or equipment) to try, and established your safe word, you're ready for your new adventure, one in which even the planning stages are part of the foreplay.

Movies and Magazines

Here's one way to start ramping up your game.

If you think of watching dirty movies as strictly a personal masturbation aid, something to engage in secretly and behind closed doors, think again. Sex for one is great, but enjoying the view with your partner can be even better. Watching an erotic film together will certainly loosen you both up and put you in the mood, but don't discount the inspiration and valuable pointers you'll get about a variety of other forbidden pleasures you've been wanting to try.

When you are planning your adult movie night, keep in mind that there are explicit films for every taste and proclivity, whether you fancy tip-to-toe leather gear, gal-on-guy penetration, exhibitionism/voyeurism, or any other form of consensual sex play. (There might even be some activities you hadn't thought of trying.) Gauge your own responses and those of your lover to the various activities you are watching, and use it as a roadmap for further exploration into virgin territory.

All of us—but especially men—get charged up by watching attractive people engaging in hot screen sex. Whether you institute a "hands off 'til it's over" policy (to add to the sexual tension), fondle and fool around during the show, or fondle yourselves—it can all be a part of your foreplay repertoire and make for great sex when the credits roll.

These days, there's no need to steal away for a visit to the local adult bookstore, either. Explicit films (classics, such as *The Devil in Miss Jones*, *Deep Throat*, *Behind the Green Door*, or my personal favorite, *The Opening of Misty Beethoven,* as well as new releases) are readily available from online stores and in specialty shops you won't be embarrassed to enter. Forget the popcorn: Soak in the film and then feast on *each other*!

There are lots of ways to heighten the fun and build the anticipation. First of all, be sure to plan your movie night ahead of time, so both of you can luxuriate in the anticipation. Picking out the movie can be part of the fun, too, if you do it together. Whether you take a joint trip to the local XXX shop or browse online together, take your time with it, pointing out the titles that particularly turn you on and taking note of your partner's specific likes and dislikes. Is he way into girl-on-girl action? Does she yearn to watch some heavy bondage and discipline? That information will come in handy on movie night as well as on future occasions, when you are catering to each other's wild fantasies or doing some of the role-playing you read about in chapter 5.

Once you've made your selection, you can have some extra fun by extending the theme of the movie to your clothing, food, and decor. Is the film about a dirty handyman and his nubile customer? A cheerleading squad and a football team? Dress up like the characters and incorporate the scenario into your own activities. A French movie might inspire a menu of Gallic snacks. Use your imagination to make your night at the movies two thumbs up all the way.

If still photos are more your style, there are gorgeous, glossy, and very sexy magazines and websites for every taste, too. For those who like to use their own imaginations to fill in the blanks, well-executed photography (the kind in this book, even can be all the guidance and superhot inspiration you need to try a new activity.

And why just look? As you are lingering over some juicy scenario or photo, take a few minutes to try out the most intriguing poses and positions yourselves, or at least discuss which things you'd like to try. As the images turn you on, don't hold back—pleasure yourself and each other with your hands, mouths, and imaginations. And don't forget about the text: Sexy magazines tend to have spicy letters and stories describing all kinds of salacious activities. Read these aloud while you fondle and finger each other to the point of distraction. The advice column is a fun place to start; once you've enjoyed the Q&A, make up some sex questions of your own and take turns providing (or demonstrating) the answers.

The trick is to enjoy the words and images together—and then create some fantasies of your own.

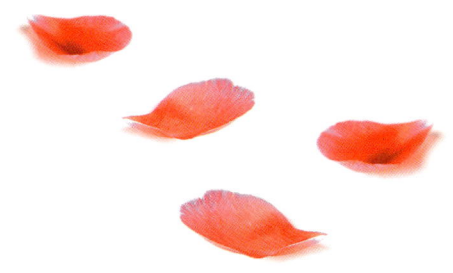

Shave and a Hair Cut

Here's a kink you might not have thought about: Certain kinds of grooming can be turn-ons in and of themselves.

Ladies, if you've never tried it, treat yourself to a Brazilian bikini wax—the kind where they remove nearly all of your pubic hair, front and back. It only stings for a few minutes, and the results can be supersexy for both of you. The look and feel of your bare vulva and pretty pink hole will drive him wild, and for you, every sensation will be enhanced. Some women say this makes them feel like prepubescent girls again, so if this sounds exciting (to you or to him), by all means book an appointment.

Men can wax too, of course, but for some reason—perhaps their lower pain threshold—many balk at the idea. No matter. Shaving each other (carefully!) can be a big turn-on, too. The process itself is exciting (set it up as your own exclusive at-home spa day) and the result is every bit as dramatic as that of a wax. Keep in mind that the grow-in can be a little itchy. But here's the good news, guys: Your penis just might look a bit bigger without its nest of pubic hair. And it might seem more inviting for oral sex, too.

When it's time for your shaving session, keep it fun and interesting. Take turns with each phase: Start by trimming each other's pubic hair, followed by slathering on the shave cream or gel (be sure to use a nonirritating kind, as you are dealing with sensitive tissues). Linger over the application of the lubricant—it will feel and smell heavenly and heighten the anticipation. When you are ready for your shave, make sure you have a comfortable spot to recline: A bed covered with towels is much more comfortable than the bathroom floor or toilet seat. And have a big bowl of warm, soapy water handy for rinsing. Use a small, swiveling multiblade razor, the kind designed "especially for women," and guide it carefully—you don't want to risk any nicks.

Once you are finished and all rinsed off, take some time to admire your handiwork. Run your fingers over your lover's delightfully nude, supersensitive skin (or take a few licks of those clean-as-a-whistle, baby-soft labia, balls, or creases). Give yourself a nice feel, too, and admire yourself in the mirror—it's like being a little kid again, but better!

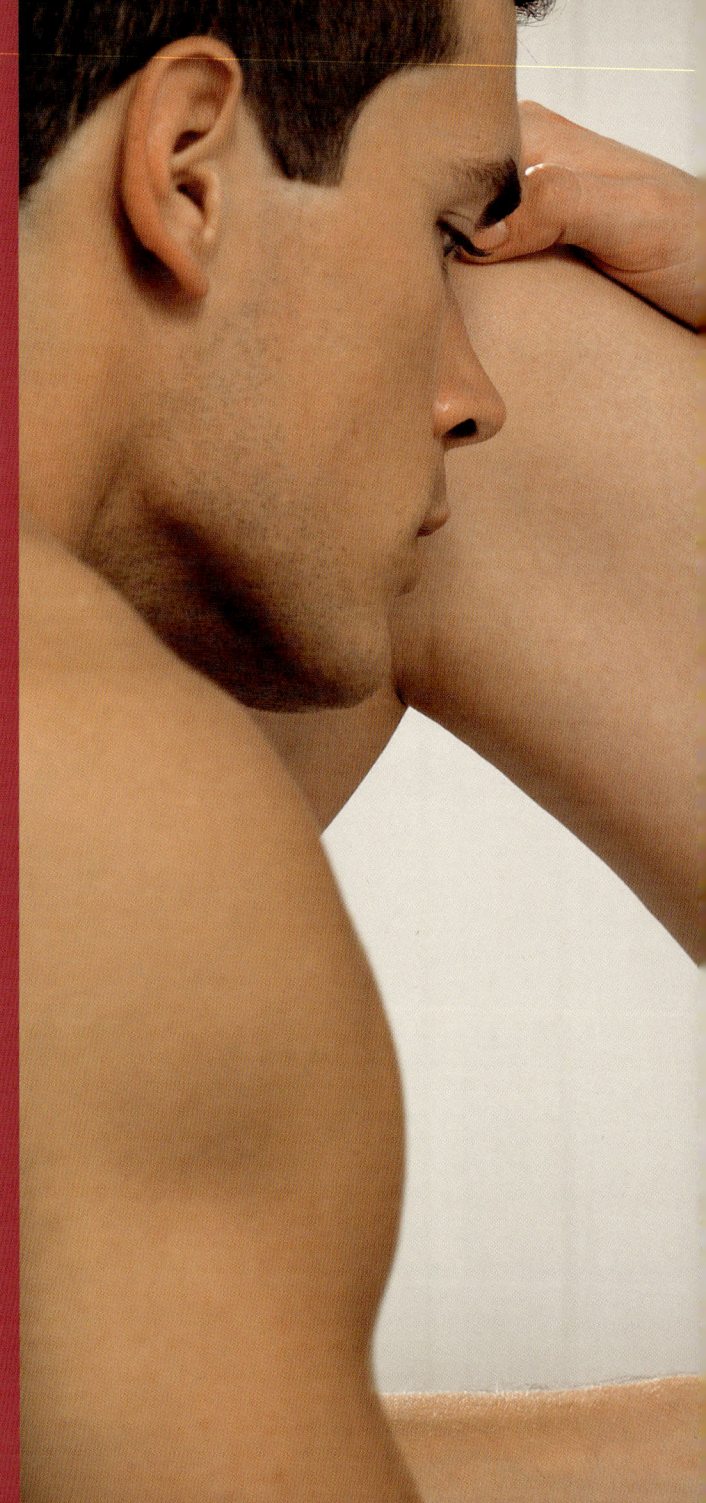

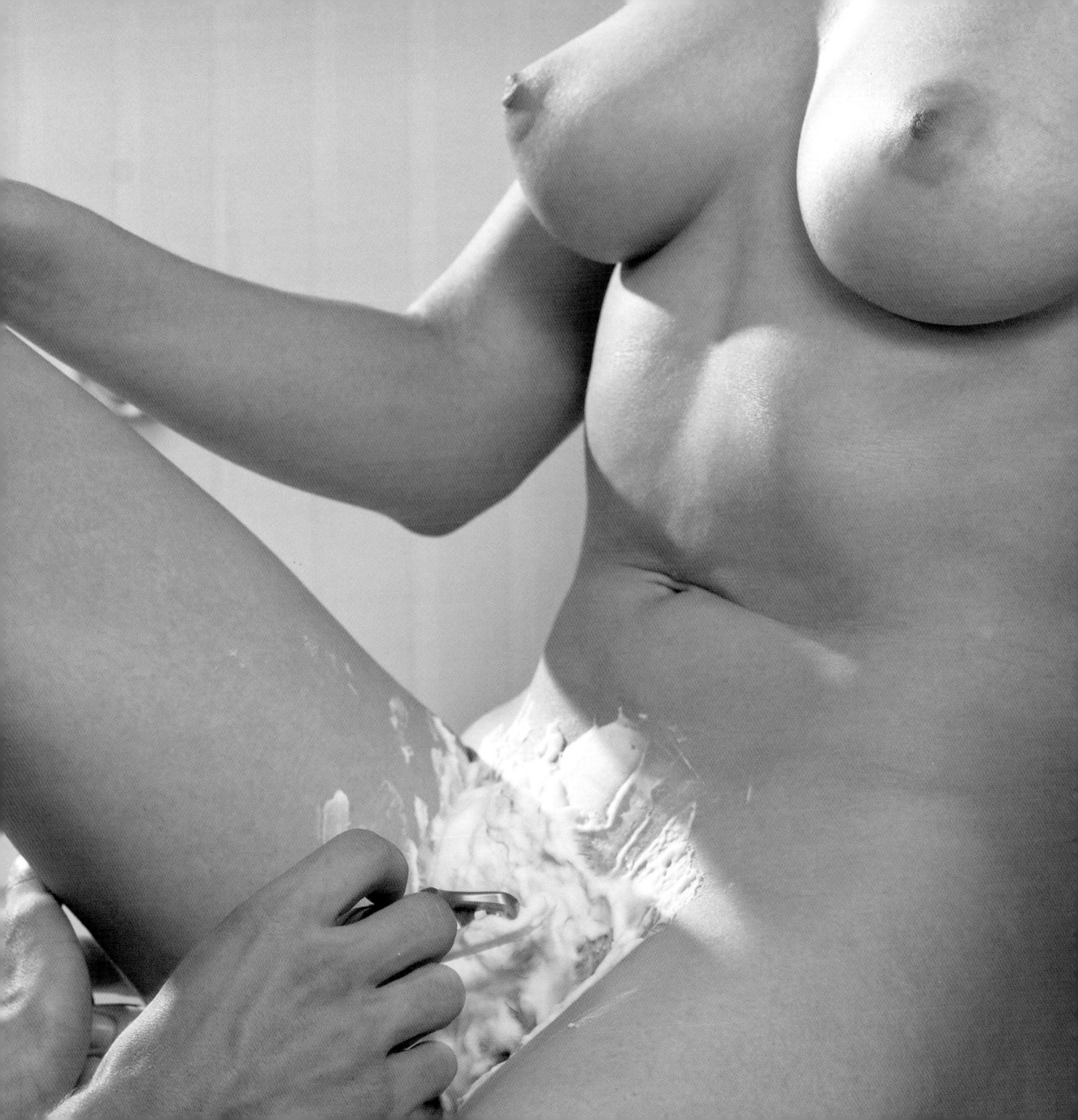

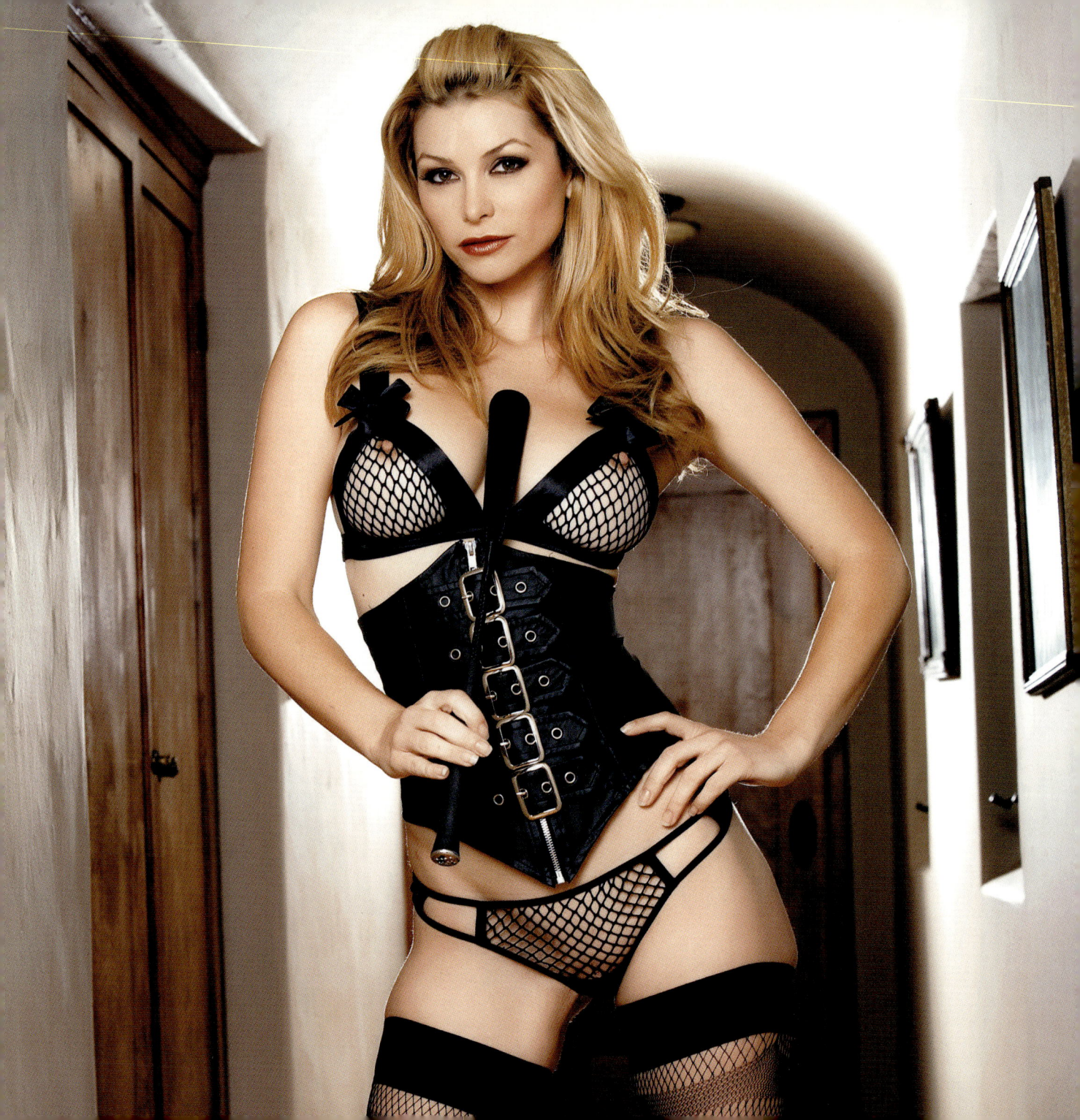

Stocks and Bondage

When you read the words "kinky sex," what's the first thing you think of? It very well might be something related to what is known as B&D, or bondage and discipline. This term has come to refer to activities involving the master-slave relationship (or boss-underling or teacher-student relationship—any relationship involving authority). It often involves restraints, special clothing, and equipment to help flesh out the master-slave fantasy. Some prefer this flavor of sexual activity above all others, but there's no reason you can't dabble in it once in a while, just for a change of pace. I guarantee that when you walk out of the bathroom in a leather bustier and thong, wearing stiletto heels, and carrying a riding crop, the foreplay will have begun in earnest.

But before we get to the really edgy stuff, let's start with the area of bondage play involving simple restraint. Here are a few moves you might want to try before you bring on the pleasurable pain:

When your lady-love comes into the room, immediately embrace and kiss her and flatter her with compliments about how beautiful and sexy she is. Sit her down comfortably, serve her a cocktail, then tell her to relax—you are going to take charge of her pleasure. Lead her to the bed and tell her to disrobe and put on the sexy lingerie you've laid out for her: lacy panties, camisole, perhaps a garter belt and stockings. When she is dressed as you've instructed, gently restrain her wrists and ankles with silk or velvet ties. Tell her that now her only responsibility is to lie back and enjoy your ministrations. Work her over slowly, fondling and caressing her breasts, sucking her nipples, and kissing your way down her abdomen and around to her buttocks, thighs, and finally her sweet pussy. The idea is to tease and tantalize her until she begs for more. The fact that she is restrained will make her feel freer than ever.

Ladies, try restraining your man as described in the previous bullet, but add a blindfold. Once you've determined that he is completely in the dark, reach into your bag of tricks and go to town on him with your favorite toys: Try those nipple clamps on him while you gently stroke his abs, ass, and thighs; insert a vibrating butt plug and then lube up his penis and give it a luxurious hand-over-hand job; drag a feather up and down the length of his torso and legs as you lick and suck his lips, ears, and neck. But if he comes close to orgasm, back off—the idea is to prolong the delicious teasing and heighten the anticipation.

Use a video camera as part of the restraint scenario and play back the results for your lover later.

Restrain and blindfold your man even more tightly this time, and tell him he is about to be worked over by a pair of beautiful twin sisters, Mona and Nina. As you work on him, make him tell you who he thinks is doing what. Is that Mona licking his balls as she massages his thighs? Is it Nina giving him upside-down kisses and dangling her breasts in his face as she massages his scalp and neck? And who is straddling his face and rubbing her beautiful mound over his mouth and nose? Try hard to do the work of two women convincingly.

Once you are ready to graduate to the hardcore stuff, decide which one of you will be the dominant lover and which one will be the submissive one for a particular session. The direction the action takes is pretty much in the hands of the dominant partner, so start giving orders. Make your slave cater to your every whim, from groveling and begging for a spanking to getting you all primed and ready for sex with an erotic all-over massage. Feel free to give orders, reward for good behavior, and "punish" for disobedience (always keeping your behavior within the boundaries you've agreed to—and stopping immediately if either of you uses the safe word or feels uncomfortable). Play your mutual roles to the hilt: Enjoy the liberation of being dominant (the freedom to go after what you want) or the equally liberating role of being submissive (the ability to relinquish all decisions to someone else and follow orders blindly, without guilt).

Here are some specific items you might want to procure and put into action on bondage night. Which of these sound hot to the two of you?

Super-High Stiletto Heels (Including Boots). Ladies, these will make you look and feel powerful when you are playing the mistress in charge. Go ahead and strut your stuff in them, and don't be afraid to make your lover kneel down and lick them clean for you. He can deny you nothing when you have him captive at the point of your shiny black boot heel!

Leather Underwear (for Both of You). Time to visit the sex boutique and pick out some racy gear to inspire your bondage play. Go together and model for each other in the dressing room—or surprise each other with some sexy gifts. You'll be amazed at the variety of garments available, from tight, lace-up bustiers and leather thongs to pointy bras, leggings, and strappy-all-over outfits that will remind you of your favorite superhero or heroine. You are sure to feel like the king and queen of the universe in black leather.

Rubber (PVC) Gear. Some prefer rubber to leather for this kind of play (though personally I find it a bit hot and confining). If it is your thing, help yourself to a skintight rubber getup (or maybe just the pants) and go to town.

Stockings, Garters, and Other Naughty Lingerie. If those slick or unnatural substances make you feel silly or uncomfortable, stick with the tried and true, but shop for something especially edgy and alluring for bondage night. Ladies, that means maybe an old-fashioned garter belt and stockings, but this time perhaps a leather garter and fishnets; a superstructured peekaboo bra with the nipples cut out, in a provocative color, along with a black leather thong that zips from front to back; a "come hither" camisole that can be laced tightly to provide maximum pressure and cleavage—the works. Crotchless panties are fun—or just wear the garter and stockings and leave the panties off altogether.

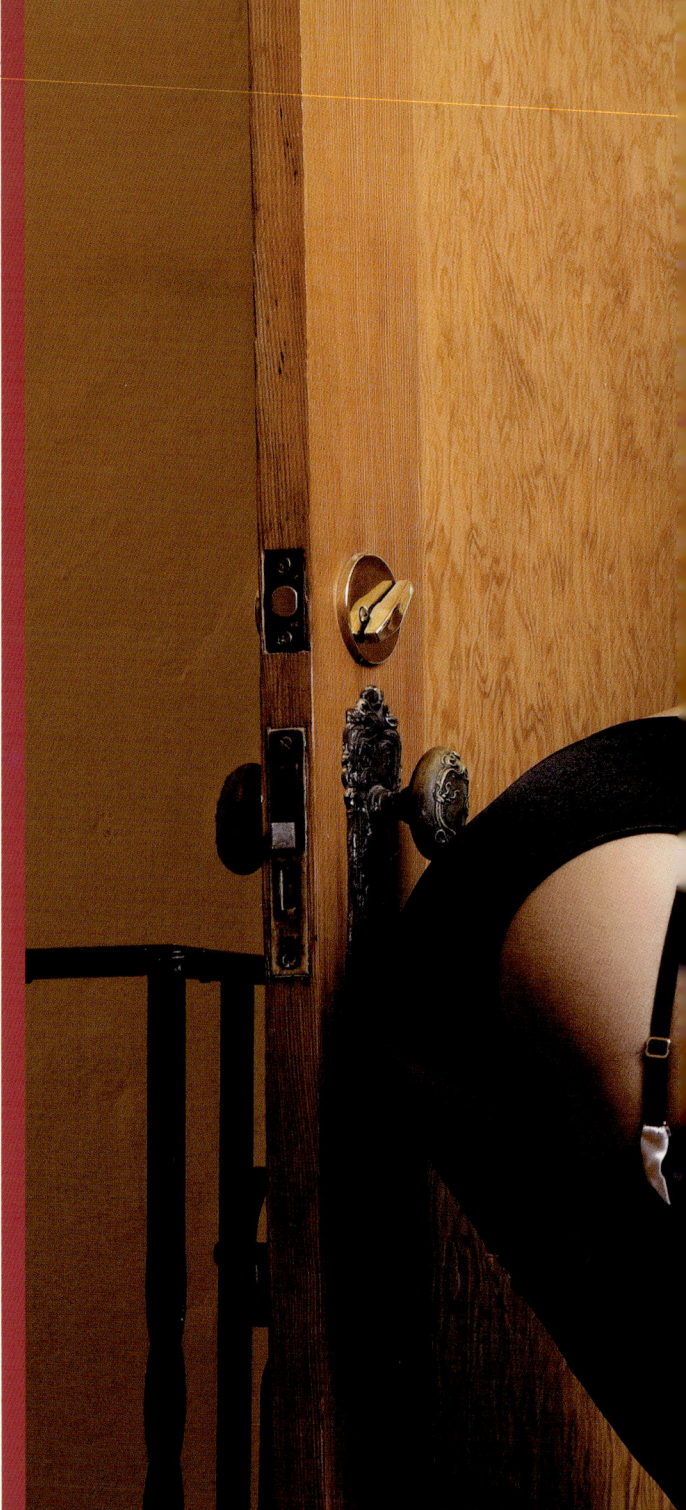

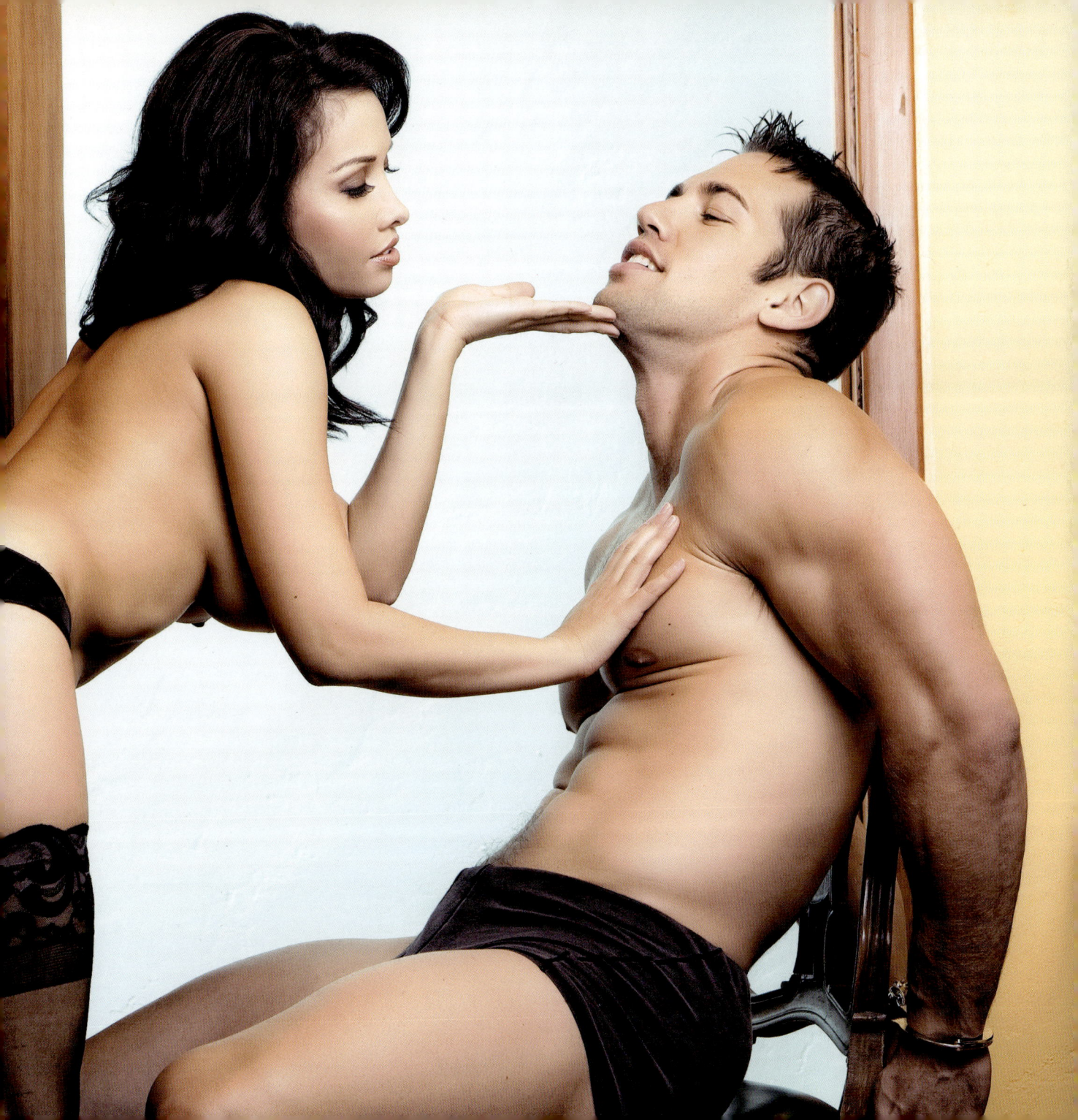

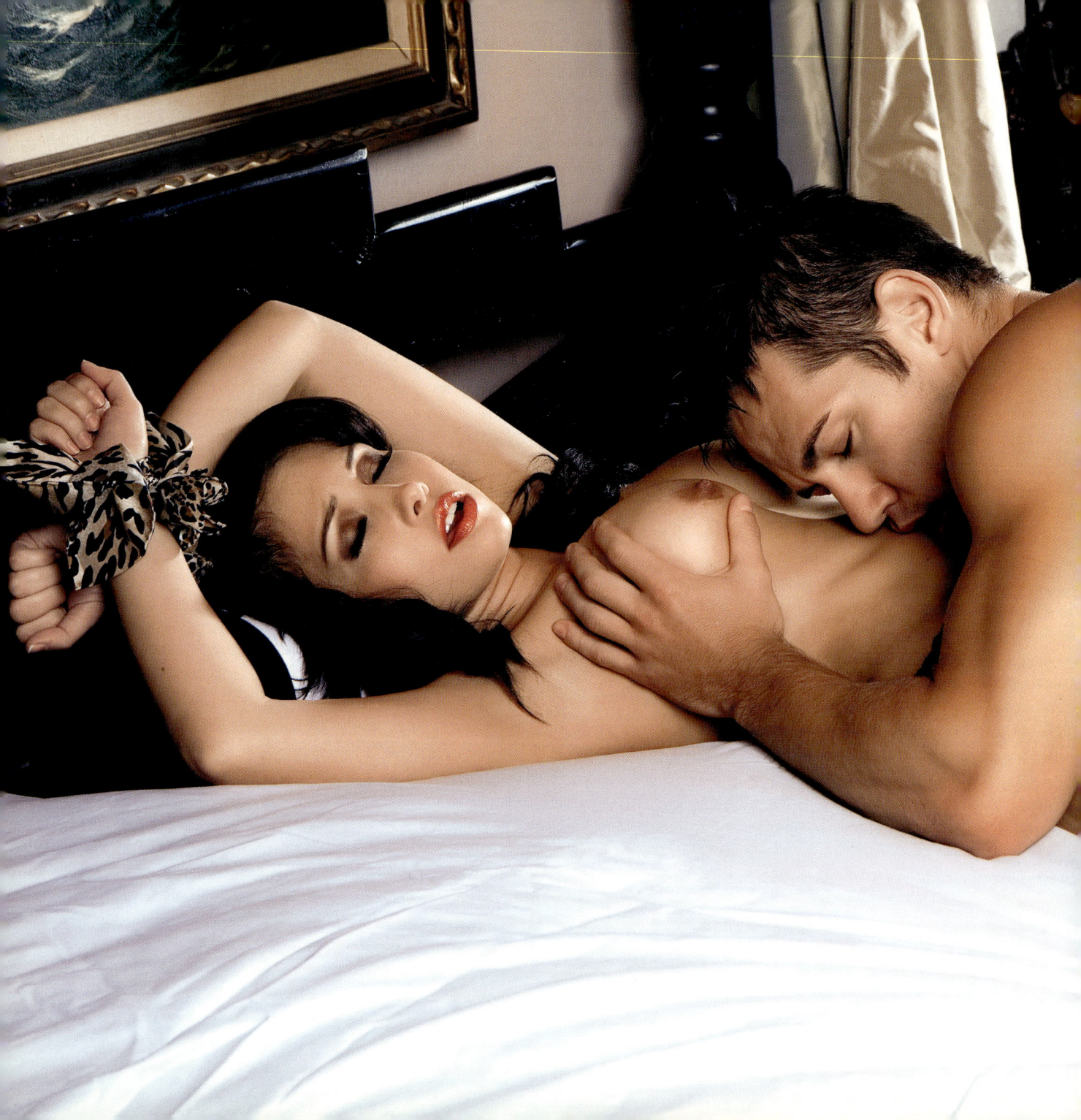

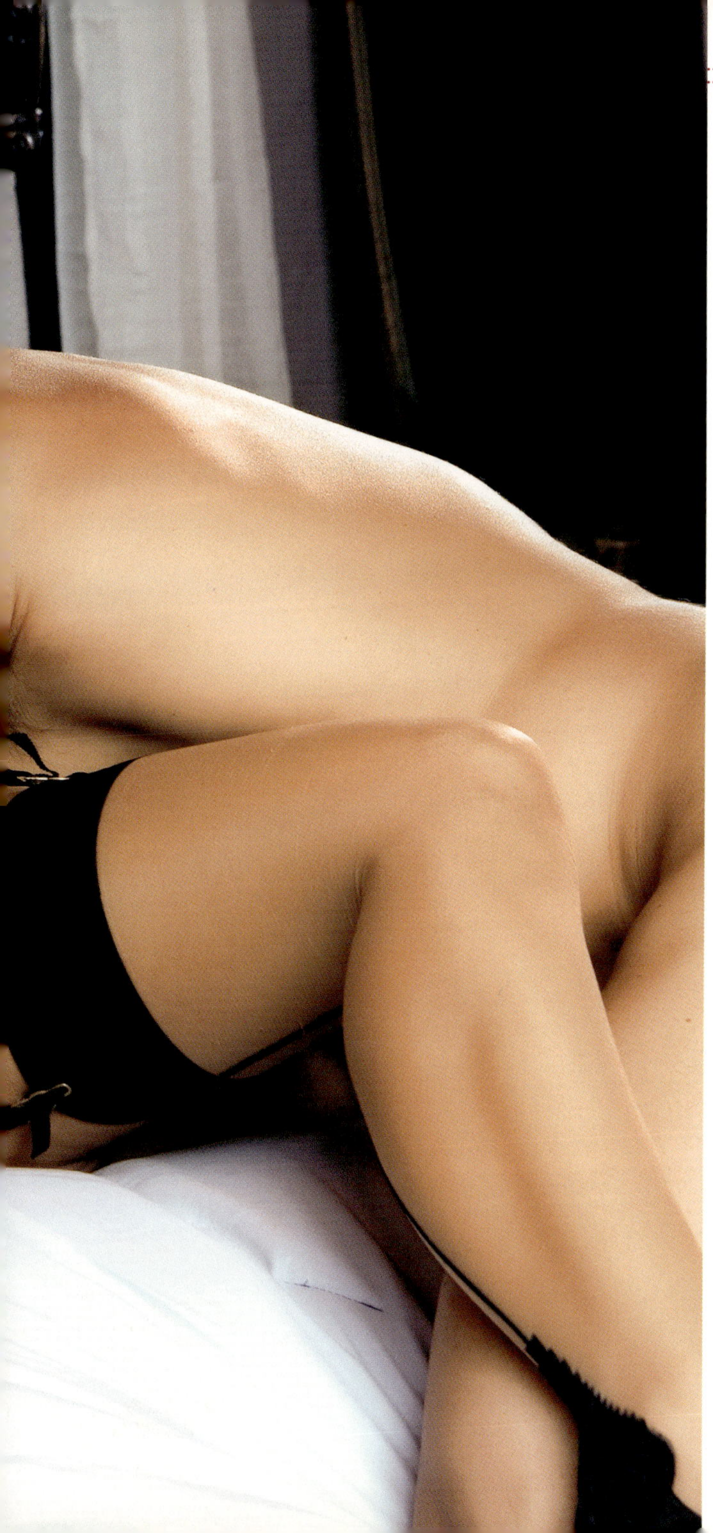

Edible undergarments can be a hoot, too (though they tend not to taste very good). Guys, for your part, try out a new kind of underwear: If you're a boxer man, try briefs, or vice versa—and be aware that they make leather underwear for you, too, complete with zippers, laces, and cutouts. At the very least, try a sexy new color and material. Black silk boxers, perhaps?

Masks and Blindfolds. As discussed earlier, masks and blindfolds are staples of bondage scenarios, and they run the gamut from the hardcore zippered leather facemask to a silk scarf tied over the eyes. Go with what makes you both feel hot, and with what helps you keep your slave in your control.

Handcuffs and Other Restraints. You've already discovered that tying up or restraining your partner can be a serious turn-on for both of you, as long as your trust and communication are strong (and you agree that either one of you can stop the show at any time). At any sex shop, you'll find handcuffs similar to those policemen use (keep the extra key somewhere safe, or get the kind with an emergency release button), as well as a variety of velvet and Velcro ties, ropes, and other items. The nicest restraints have lined wrist or ankle bands to guard against rope burns and abrasions. If you decide to improvise with what you have in the house (twine, duct tape, etc.), be mindful of these kinds of injuries.

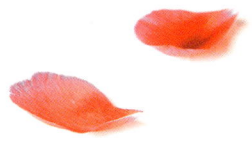

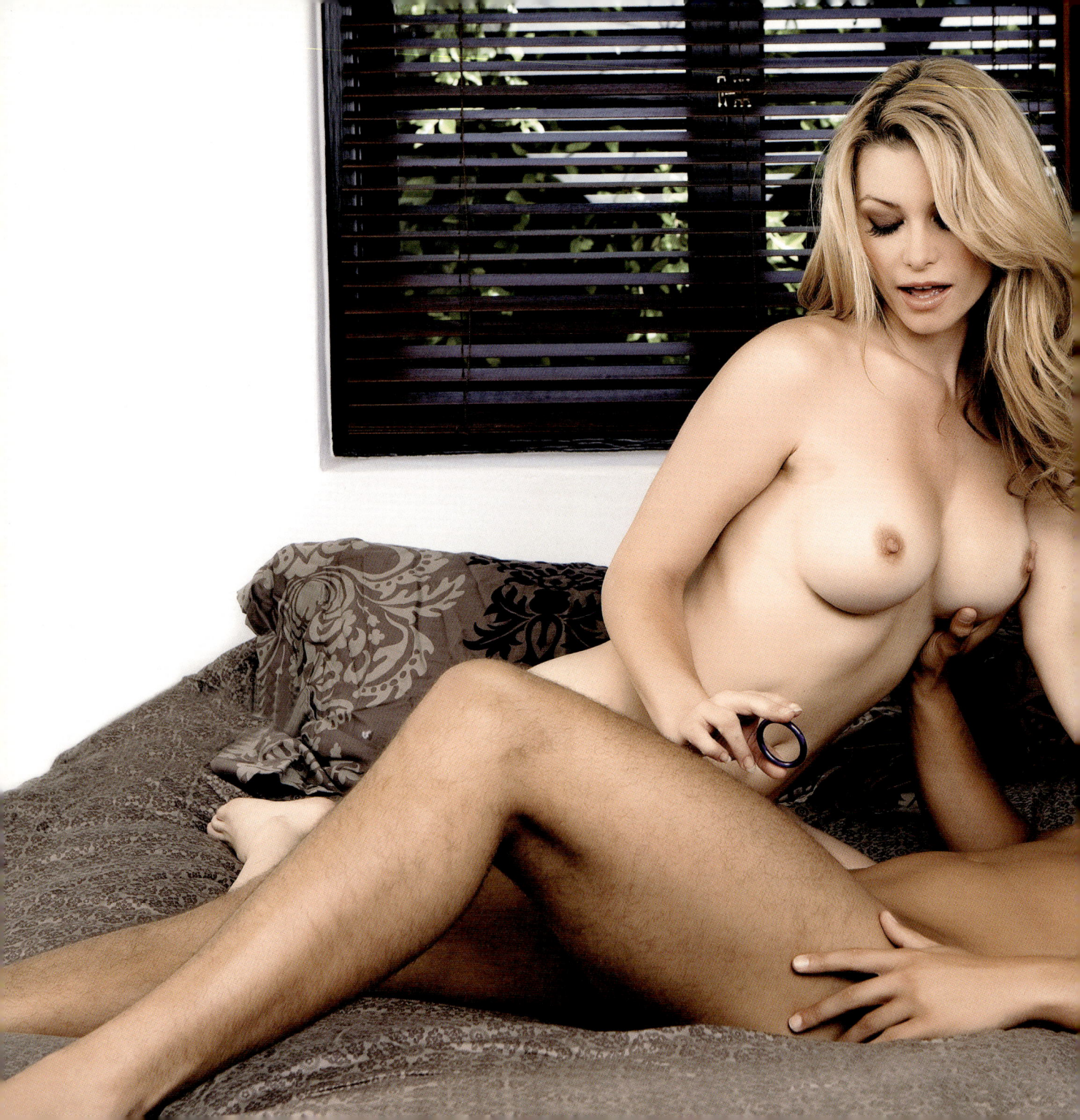

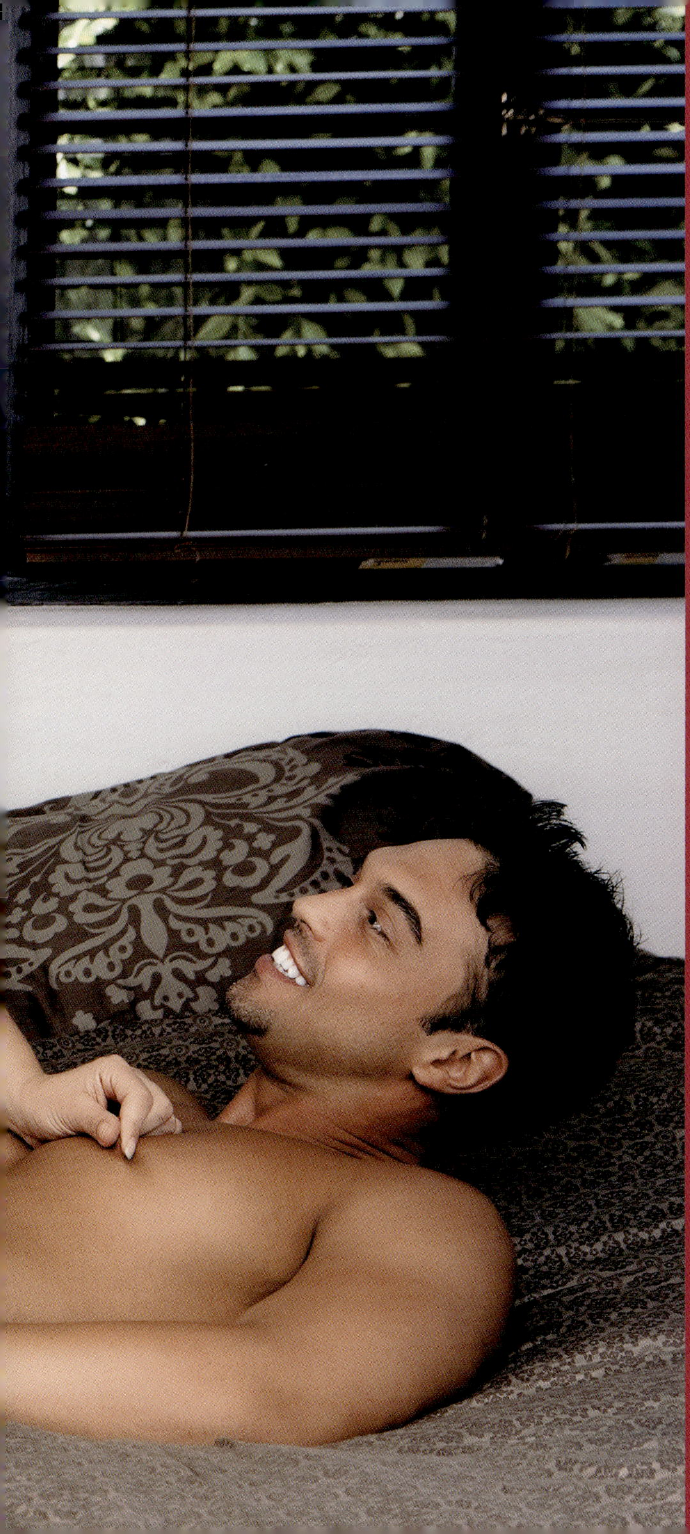

Cock Rings. Many men just love the tight feeling they get from wearing a cock ring and say they get their biggest erections when they are wearing one. (Though they are called *cock* rings, most are designed to go around the balls as well.) Ladies, let him pick out the one he wants, and don't be shy about asking a salesclerk for guidance. The most popular ones are made of either leather and snaps or metal, and they are usually adjustable for maximum comfort. Extra thrills for *both* of you can be had with a vibrating cock ring, designed to stimulate a lady's clitoris and a man's scrotum simultaneously. Here's a personal tip: Ladies, once the two of you own a cock ring, come to dinner some night (at home or at a restaurant) wearing it around your wrist. Your man will get the hint immediately, and I promise you he will *race* through dinner to get to the next phase of the evening!

Nipple Clamps. Both men and women can wear nipple clamps—and the exquisite pain they cause can be a thrill (. . . or not, so experiment and feel free to say "No, thanks" if you are too sensitive to enjoy them). These can be a great accoutrement to a discipline scenario: If she is a bad girl, just give those clamps a tweak. Start with them on the loose side, then keep tightening to the point where they feel just right.

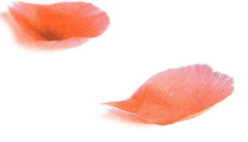

Whips, Crops, and Spankers. What do you do with a naughty, naughty girl? Give her a spanking, that's what. If you both agree to this behavior, and agree to stop if it's too much, there are all kinds of implements to use (besides your bare palms, of course) to inflict a little rear-end correction. Check out the crops, whips, and other spanking devices at your local sex shop—or use a real riding crop. Paddles, hairbrushes, or even a rolled up magazine can work, as well. Just be humane to your lover and make sure that even in the heat of the moment your brute force is at least 75 percent acting. She will let you know if she wants more.

Hot Wax. If you've ever accidentally dripped candle wax on yourself, you know that it burns for a second—but after that, it feels kind of . . . nice. You might want to experiment with candle wax during foreplay, for that lovely momentary pain, followed by excellent warmth. Be careful of getting it near your more sensitive areas, such as sex organs or nipples. The back, abdomen, or limbs are the best spots for administering this kind of "punishment."

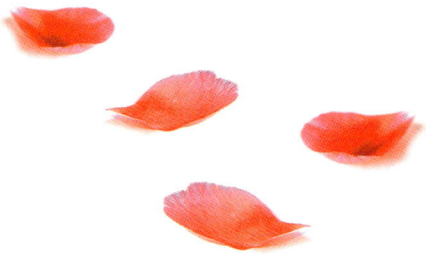

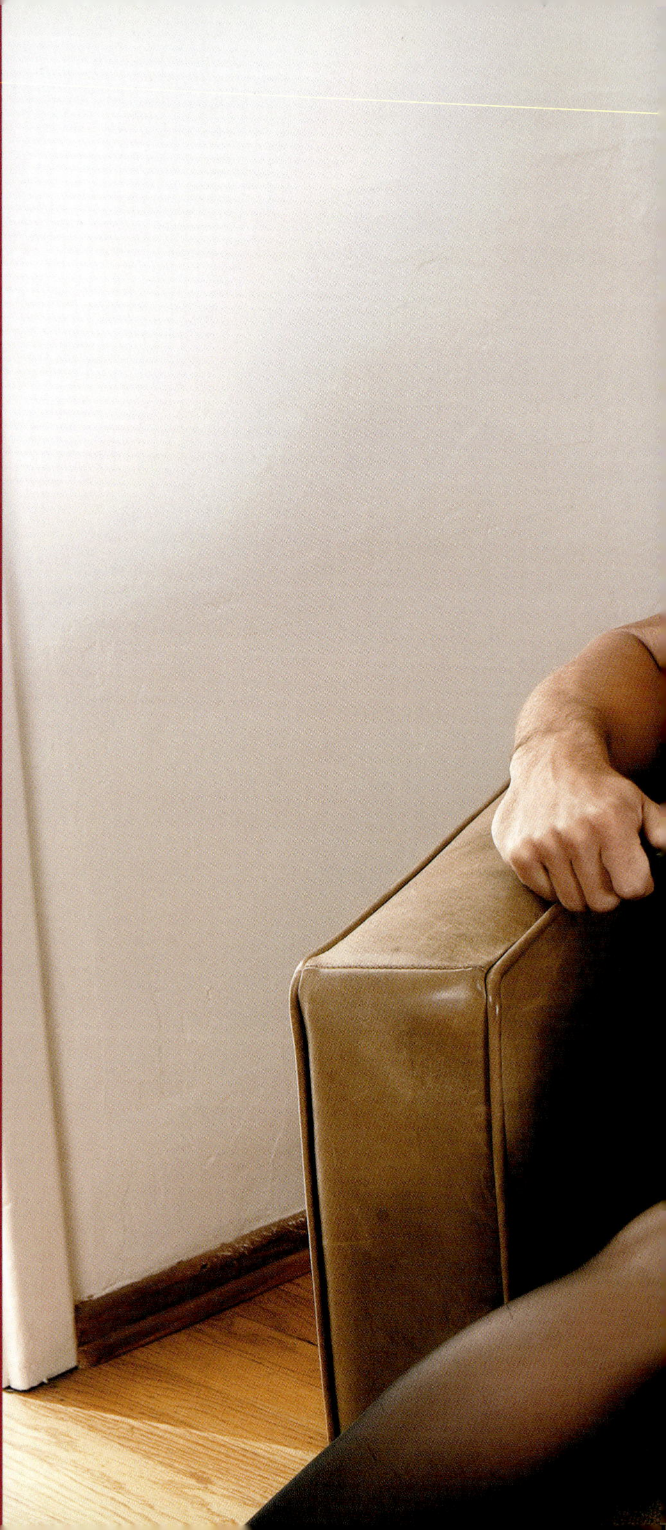

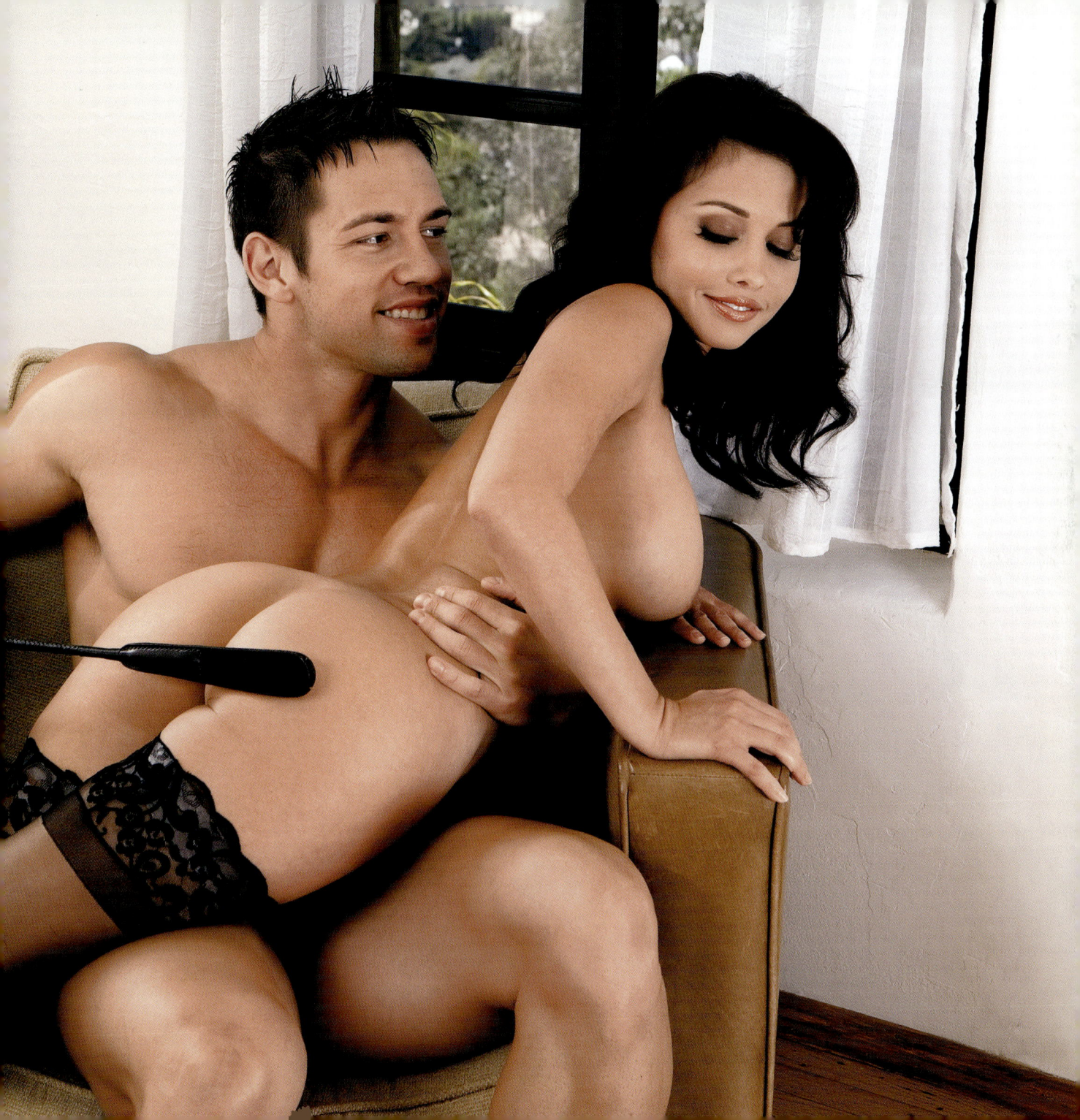

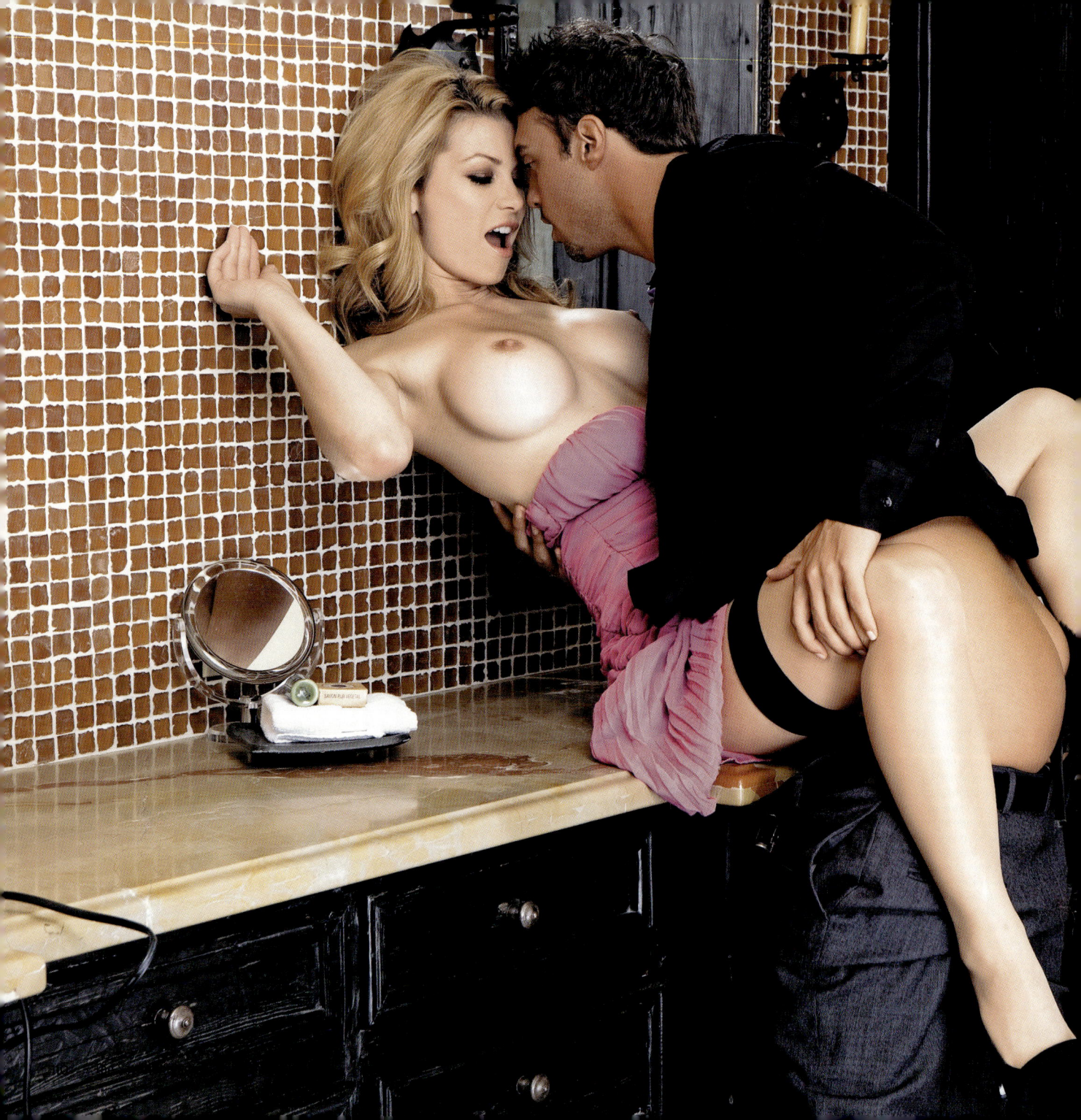

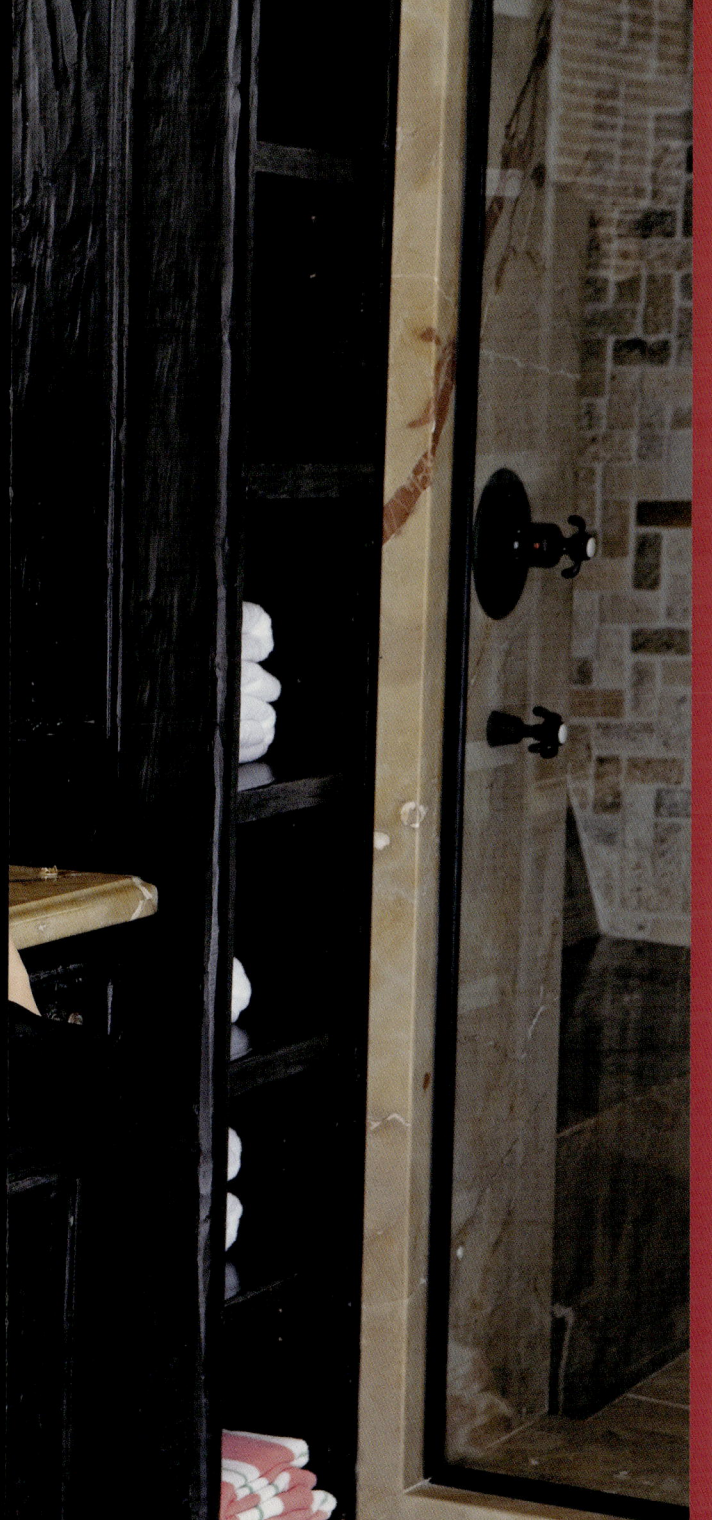

Peekaboo!

Let's talk about a few other "outside the lines" practices that might pique your interest. Have you ever fantasized about showing the world your most private acts? Lots of people get off on exhibiting themselves or their lovers. If you think that might be your thing (or might turn your lover on), start by leaving the lights on and the curtains and shades *open* one night. As you kiss, fondle, and caress each other, imagine who might be watching and how they might respond. Is your neighbor across the street masturbating while he watches your woman stroke your hard cock? What would he think if you pinned her backside against the window and had your way with her?

Another way to fulfill those exhibitionist fantasies is to engage in sexual activity in public or "high-risk" places, where there is a chance you might get caught. This could include the upstairs bedroom at a friend's dinner party, the bathroom on an airplane, or the backseat of a cab. For more on this particular thrill, check out chapter 8.

Voyeurism is the flip side of exhibitionism. Voyeurs would rather watch the action than participate—and a free show can be enjoyable for all of us once in a while. Try performing for one another or engaging in a little bit of "Peeping Tom" activity if you have a chance. (Do your neighbors ever leave *their* shades open? They might just be begging for an audience.) If you or your lover has a penchant for watching, you can set up scenarios where you secretly watch each other from hidden vantage points. Maybe you even want to go outside and look in your own window while your lover masturbates. (If you confine these games to yourselves, you won't have to worry about what to say when you run into your neighbors at the grocery store.)

Can I Borrow That Slip?

Cross-dressing isn't for everyone, but don't knock it until you've tried it. It can be very exciting for both men and women to shed their own identities and try on their mate's—right down to the panties. Ladies, seriously: You haven't lived until you've worn a pair of his jockeys (feel free to stuff them for the full effect!) Try the suit and tie, too—the works! And gentlemen, a pair of stockings and high heels can be enormously empowering in the privacy of your bedroom. And if even that is too much, try simply wearing a pair of her silk panties to work one day, under your street clothes. That tiny little secret could keep you hot all day!

Like all high-risk activities, trust between you is key, and the result will be a deeper bond and greater mutual insight.

Bag of Tricks

It's time to delve more deeply into sex toys.

Maybe you own a dildo or vibrator (most of us have purchased one at some point) and think of it as your substitute when there's no lover in sight. It's true that they can be helpful in the self-love department—but what about adding some toys to your foreplay routine? Just because there's a real penis in the room doesn't mean you can't introduce a lovely synthetic one to the scenario. Think of the whole range of sensations and simultaneous (or alternative) stimulation you can explore, with the help of your little mechanical or silicone friends.

There is a wide variety of vibrators, dildos, and other devices on the market (available at sex shops and online specialty stores), and there are whole books on the subject of using them, including the extremely enlightening (and sexy!) *Big Book of Sex Toys*, by Tristan Taormino. To get you started and open your mind to the introduction of toys into your foreplay repertoire, here's the lowdown on my favorite toys and tools.

Dildos and More Dildos

Though the origin of the term *dildo* is unclear (among other theories, some believe it is a corruption of the Italian word *diletto*, or delight), they have clearly been around since ancient times. If you've shopped for dildos, then you know that nowadays, they come in literally hundreds of shapes, sizes, colors, and materials, with a whole host of twists. My bottom line on dildos: Check out the silicone rubber ones (though they cost a bit more than PVC)—or even the solid glass or chrome-plated steel models, if you like that sense of rigidity and hardness. Find the size and shape that's right for you and decide how lifelike you want it to be (some look more like penises than penises do)—and don't shy away from the variations, including these:

Dildo with Harness. These are designed to be strapped on so that a woman can anally penetrate or "peg" her man—or penetrate another woman, of course. Some of these include an external vibrator for the benefit of the wearer. Ladies, you haven't lived until you've strapped one on, even if you don't end up going the distance with your guy. The sense of power you'll feel (and wait until you look in the mirror!) is one of the great turn-ons. Go ahead and stroke yourself! If you think the sight of this will dampen the fun for your lover, however, save it for a private moment.

Double-Ended Dildo. It's just what it sounds like, and serves the obvious purpose: the double model can be used from both sides simultaneously, by two women or by a woman who wants to penetrate her man anally while being penetrated herself. This one opens up a range of possibilities that might just be right for you. If so, give it a whirl. Just be careful not to overestimate the size that will be comfortable for both of you, and go slowly and gently.

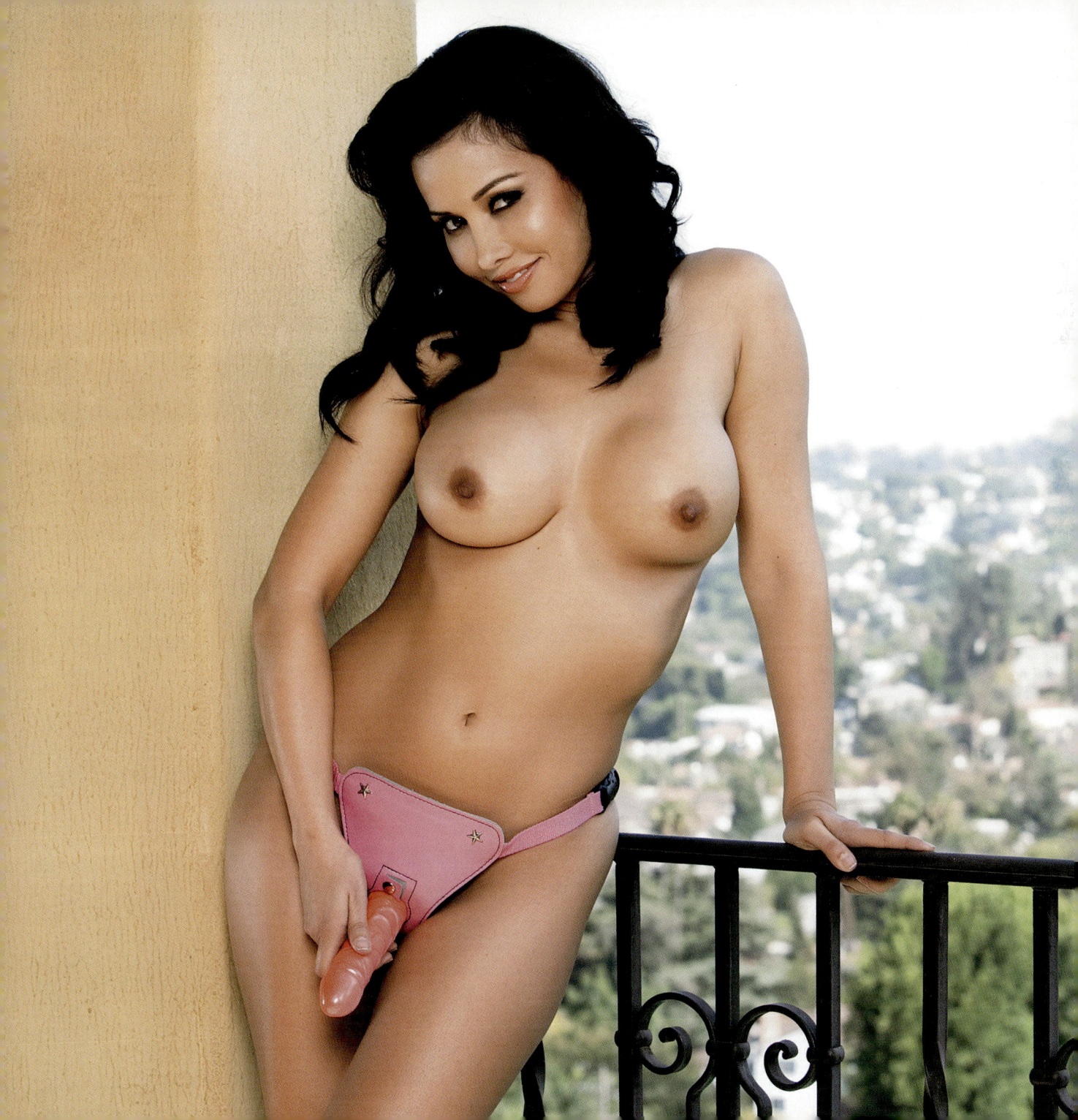

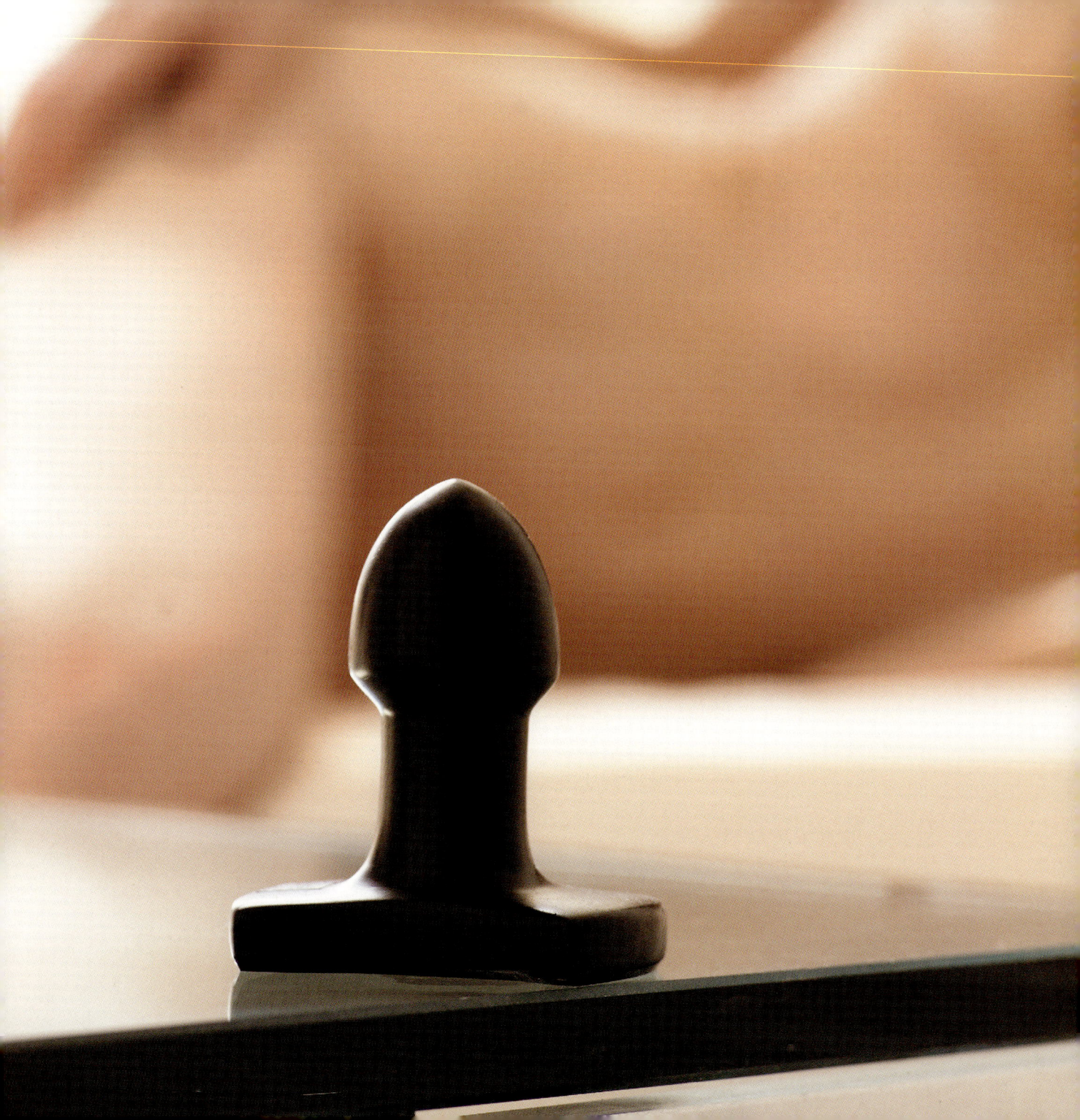

No Sex, Please

While we're dwelling in the extra-credit world of edgy foreplay, here's something unconventional to try: a sex ban. This is particularly useful if you feel your sex play has gotten a bit stale, or if you aren't fooling around as frequently as you'd both like.

Between you, decide on a period during which you agree *not* to have sex. It can be a few days, a week, a month—but make sure it is a sufficiently lengthy period of time to make you miss it.

It's uncanny. The minute you decide to forego something, there's nothing you want more! Feel free to tease each other, even fondle and pleasure each other up to a point—but no orgasms and no penetration. Try it and you'll understand that withholding sex can be the sexiest thing imaginable. And when you finally do lift that ban, you are bound to have the best sex of your lives.

There are other ways to apply this idea to foreplay, without instituting an all-out ban. The power of *withholding* touch can be just as strong as the power of touch itself. Women respond particularly well to this tactic, often reaching orgasm even as they beg to feel your hands or mouth on them. As you find the pace of your foreplay quickening, slow it down. *S-l-o-w it dooooowwwwwwnnnnnn.* Lighten your touch to the point where your lover can barely feel your hands or mouth. Resort to using your breath alone. And when things are getting very hot and heavy, just *stop* for a few seconds or even a few minutes. Hands off.

Varying the pace this way can prolong your lovemaking, deepen its intensity—and definitely make it more memorable. In the heat of the moment, don't forget the tremendous power of . . . doing nothing.

Butt Plug. (See photo, opposite.) Here's a dildo designed specifically for anal penetration—a better bet than the double for that purpose. It is designed to fit snugly inside the anus and can then be sat upon, pushed, twisted, and manipulated, or simply left in place to provide a delicious feeling of tightness and stimulation.

Wall-Mount Dildo. These don't have much to do with foreplay, unless your man gets off on watching you use one. (I bet he will!) They come with heavy-duty suction cups so they can be attached to any flat surface and used solo.

Vibrating (or Oscillating) Dildo. The best of these buzzing beauties include a way to remove the vibrator altogether in order to clean it thoroughly. How could you not enjoy a session that includes simultaneous penetration and vibration or oscillation (a swinging motion)? Let your man wield the instrument of pleasure, and he'll be over the moon just watching your face and listening to your moans and sighs.

Dildo Kit. Guys, do you want to create an exact replica of your own erect penis and present it to your mate? There are kits available for this purpose. Think of it as the gift that keeps on giving!

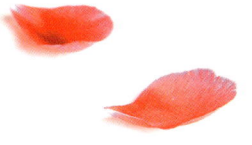

Good Vibrations

There are as many variations on vibrators as there are on dildos (and many combinations of the two), so shop, ask questions, and select something suited to your personal pleasure style. Here are a few to try:

Fingertip (or Full Glove) Vibrator. He definitely won't mind slipping *this* onto his finger! These delicate little buzzers can be used to target very specific areas, including the nipples, perineum, anus, and clitoris. The glove variation gives you a whole handful of vibes and lots of control.

Bullet or Egg. These are shaped just as they are named, fit nicely into the palm of your hand, and usually have a variety of intensity settings. (See bullet vibe in photo, right.)

Rabbit. Yes, the device made famous by *Sex and the City*. These ingenious lifesavers are designed with two "ears" to stimulate both the vagina and clitoris simultaneously. Again, let your man wield it for you (you might have to show him how) and he'll feel very much a part of the action—and a source of your pleasure.

Just for Him. There are vibrators designed specifically for men's pleasure. They often have a harness to hold them in place over the penis and testicles and can be used during sex as well as foreplay (the vibrations will stimulate both of you).

G-Spot Stimulator. The "come here," crooked-finger shape is designed specifically to stimulate the G-spot; experiment with different levels of intensity to find the one that drives you into the stratosphere.

There's an App for That. It's true. There is a bullet-shaped vibrator designed to activate when you receive a mobile phone call or text. Strap it on, and your lover can control your pleasure by ringing your chimes!

Now that you are familiar with the equipment, here are some ideas for using it for mad-hot foreplay:

First, make sure you've set the scene for fun. As a change of pace from the bedroom, create a love nest in the living room with fluffy blankets and throws. Dress in your naughtiest gear, light some candles, and surprise him when he walks in the door. Keep the toys out of sight, in a velvet bag or under a blanket, so you can take him by surprise as things heat up. (This is assuming you've both agreed that this kind of play is a turn-on.)

Once he is undressed and comfy, cover him with kisses and then tell him you are in charge for the evening and you plan to use all of the tools at your disposal to bring him pleasure. Then, one by one, bring out your sex toys and put them into action.

Start with a dildo and demonstrate it on yourself, first teasing yourself with its tip and then inserting it inside you and playing with it. Show him how much pleasure this is giving you—then make him lick your juices off of it. When it is all clean, tell him you are going to use it on him and try some anal play, keeping his comfort threshold in mind.

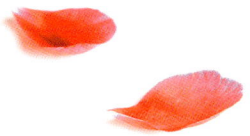

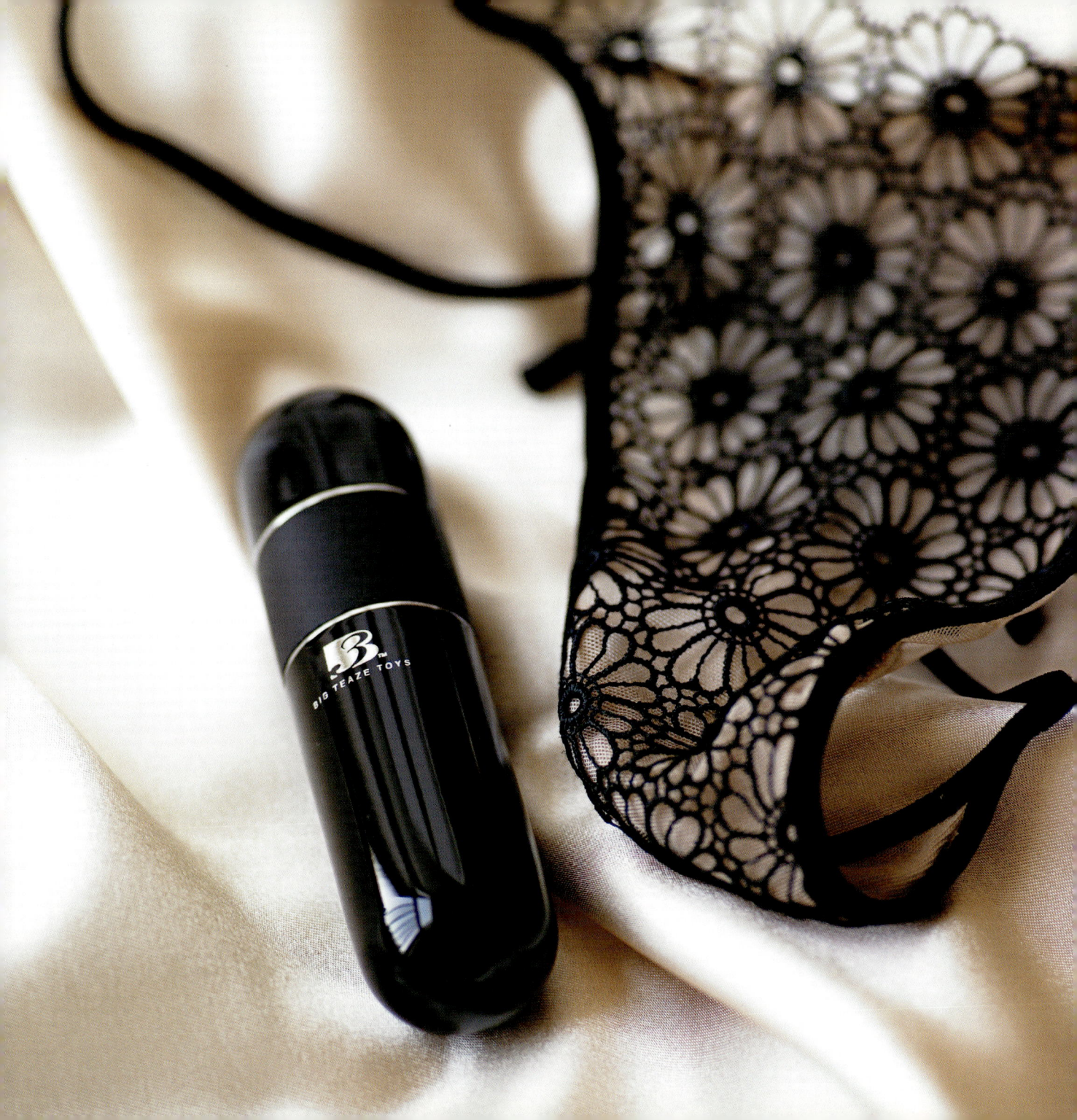

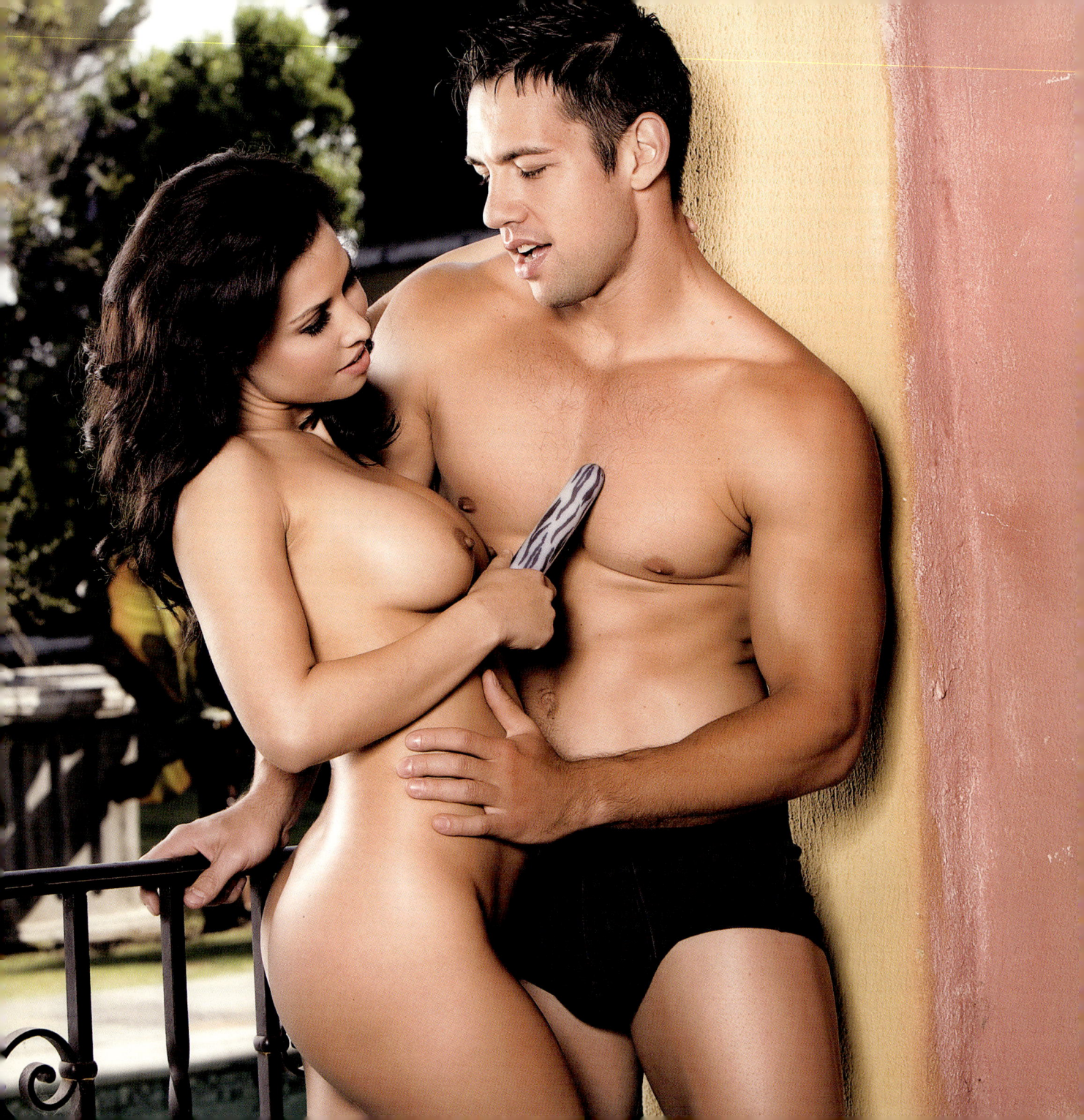

Next, take out a vibrator and use it to massage his neck and shoulders. Move on to his abdomen, paying special attention to his nipples, and gradually work your way down to his penis and balls, buzzing all the way. (Those vibrating gloves are fantastic on nipples!) Feel free to take a turn pleasuring yourself; watching you writhe with pleasure will be as sexy to him as the feeling of the vibe all over his body.

Next, lube up, insert a butt plug, and go to town on his penis, stroking it with your bare hands or with a vibrating device. Throughout your session, do your best to keep him from coming; if you think he's nearing climax, move on to the next device. Tell him he needs your permission to come—and then give it to him when you think he is ready to burst!

If your man's mind (and ass) are fully open to anal play, take it up a level. Lube up the strap-on and give it to him up the ass like the strong and sexy back-door woman you are! Just be prepared to take the bottom position when your turn comes.

For a variation, add a blindfold and make him guess which device you are using, or tie him up so he has no choice but to let you do all of the work.

To get your spankers into the act, tell him you are going to ask him a series of questions. If he answers correctly, he will get a reward (perhaps a sip of champagne or a grape, or just a delicious kiss). For every incorrect answer, though, he receives punishment: a spank, slap, or swat with one of the implements you have for the purpose.

Cock rings or any of these toys can be demonstrated on your lover (and on yourself while he watches) as part of foreplay. Don't forget to try multiple toys at once, and use those vibrating devices all over his body. Keep him guessing and begging for more.

This list is for starters. Now let your own fantasies take over and let the tools and equipment inspire you beyond the conventional, to new heights. Nothing is off-limits if you communicate, trust, and open your minds to one another's whims and fantasies. You'll be a stronger, happier couple for it—and a well-satisfied one.

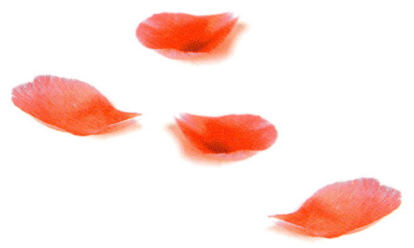

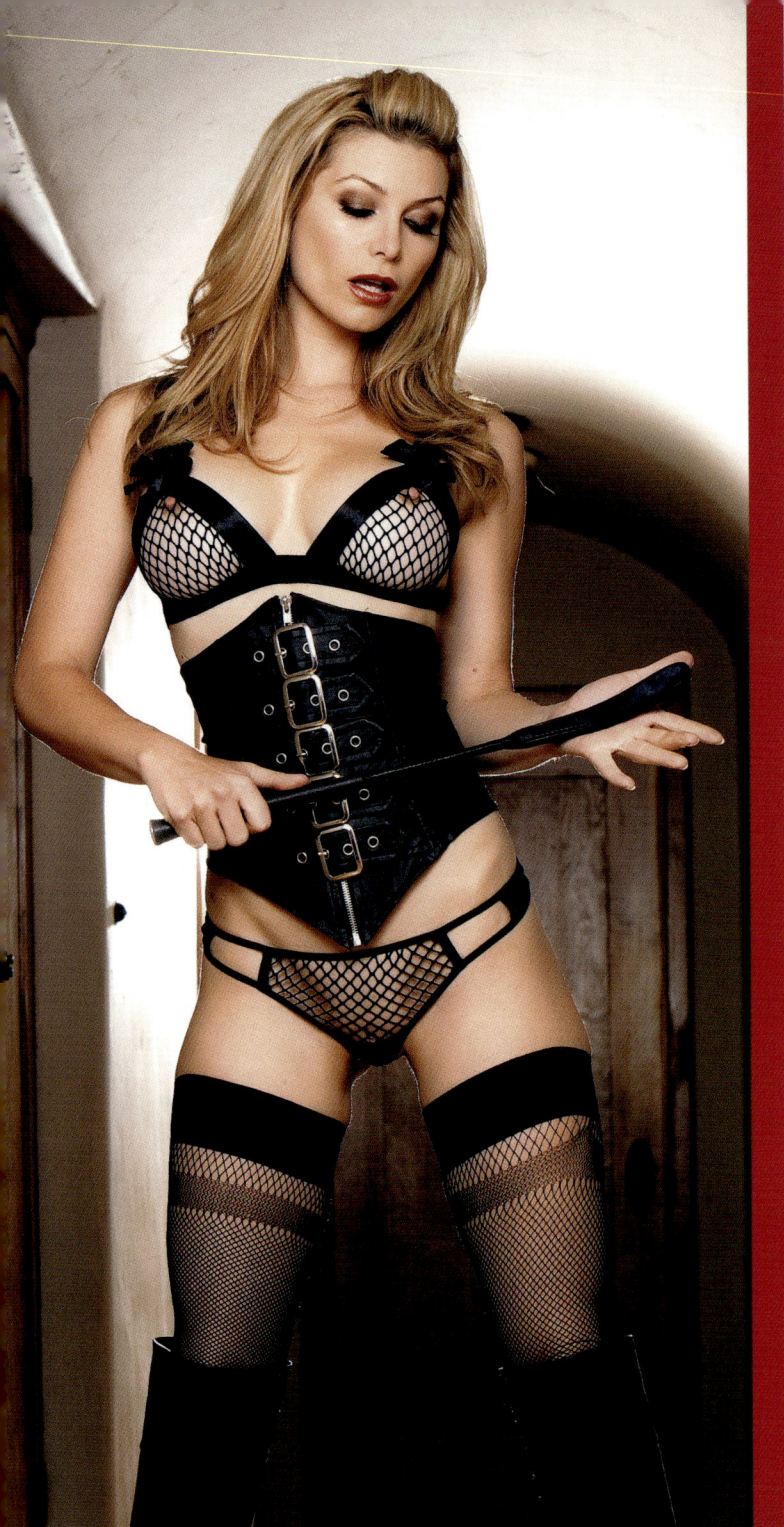

Why They Call It ForePLAY: Six Sexy Games That Will Bring Out the Beast in Both of You!

Tell Me a Story. You probably played some version of this as a kid—but now you are old enough for the X-rated version. Get comfortable and let your imagination roam free. One of you should grab an object (a stuffed animal, seashell—whatever you find handy). Holding the object signifies that you have the floor. Start telling a story that you make up on the spot. Make it realistic, set in familiar surroundings, or make it a wild fantasy. It can start out innocently enough, but leave room for it to go in an adventurous, sexy direction. Once you've got the ball rolling, pass the object to your partner, signifying that it is his or her turn to continue. As you take turns, keep trying to top each other with hotter, sexier scenes designed to turn your lover on. Which of you has the naughtier imagination? Don't be surprised to find that both of your wildest sex fantasies come out of hiding during the course of the game. Soon you may be enacting the very scenes you've described!

Love Deck. This one takes a little more preparation. Divide a pack of index cards in half, and each of you take some time to write down your sexual wishes, one per card. These should be things your mate can help you fulfill—anything from "I'd like my lover to make me come while we are in a public place" to "I'd like my lover to answer the door naked" to "I'd like to experience a half hour of nonstop oral pleasuring." Try to think of at least a dozen wishes each. Then shuffle your two sets of cards together. Now you have a love deck to use any time you desire. When you want to spice up your lovemaking, just pick a card and live the fantasy. If you want to be fair and take turns, color code your cards—pink for girls, blue for boys.

Strip *Anything*. You've heard of strip poker, but any game can incorporate the doffing of clothes into its official playbook. Even Scrabble! If that's your game, just add this option: You can trade in one tile in exchange for one piece of clothing. In checkers, every "king" can mean a clothing item comes off. (Just be sure you keep the room warm enough to be comfortable in.)

The Mirror Game. This one is designed to bring you closer. You may have noticed that touch is hotter when you are really locked in to each other, and that starts with eye contact. Though it can feel strange to stare into someone's eyes (we are taught that staring is rude, after all), it can be a beautiful way to connect more fully during foreplay and sex. To practice locking eyes, play this useful game. Sit opposite each other and stare into each other's eyes, without glancing away for even a second. Gradually, start to move in unison, with one of you taking the lead and the other mirroring his or her moves. Move slowly and deliberately, mirroring each move exactly, without ever releasing your gaze. (If you are really in tune, someone watching you won't be able to tell who is leading and who is following.) Take turns leading. Once you've mastered this, move on to a touch variation, where you are mirroring each other's caresses. Mmm!

Cold Sex. This one owes its origins to the Tantric tradition, and has nothing to do with the temperature in the room. The idea is to make an appointment with your lover to have sex at a certain time and place—and then just DO it. No soul-revealing conversations, no compliments, no caresses or sweet embraces: just quick, hot coupling. (In this case, *foreplay* means no foreplay at all!) Believe it or not, this can be incredibly exciting, especially if you and your mate have been together for a long time. It is almost like having sex with a stranger, or as a professional obligation—a fantasy for many women *and* men. Of course you don't want the remoteness to last too long, so cuddle afterward and share your thoughts about this wham-bam experience.

No Touch. We'll end with a very challenging one—but trust me, it's not impossible! This is a concentration game that is meant to bring you as close together as two people can be. The idea is to bring each other to orgasm without touching each other (or yourselves) *at all*. Use only your thoughts, concentration, eye contact, and language. To make it a little easier, you can use your breath on each other—but no hands, mouths, or anything else. In the Tantric tradition, when you look into your lover's eyes just as he or she is coming, it is called "soul gathering" and is said to help form an unbreakable bond. If you can soul gather without the benefit of physical contact, you have reached a pinnacle of lovemaking prowess.

Part III:
Exploreplay

Beyond the Bedroom: Fun with Water

Let's get wet—all over. Baths, showers, hot tubs, midnight swims in an ocean or a lake . . . all of these can become the setting for satisfying sex play, for those times when you feel like being clean and dirty at the same time! Here are a few ideas for working H_2O into your S-E-X.

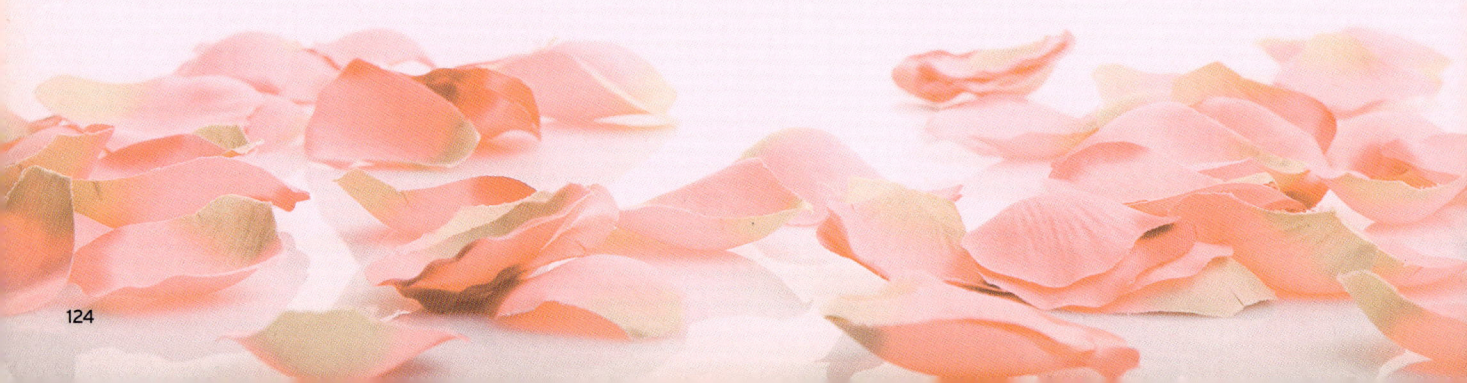

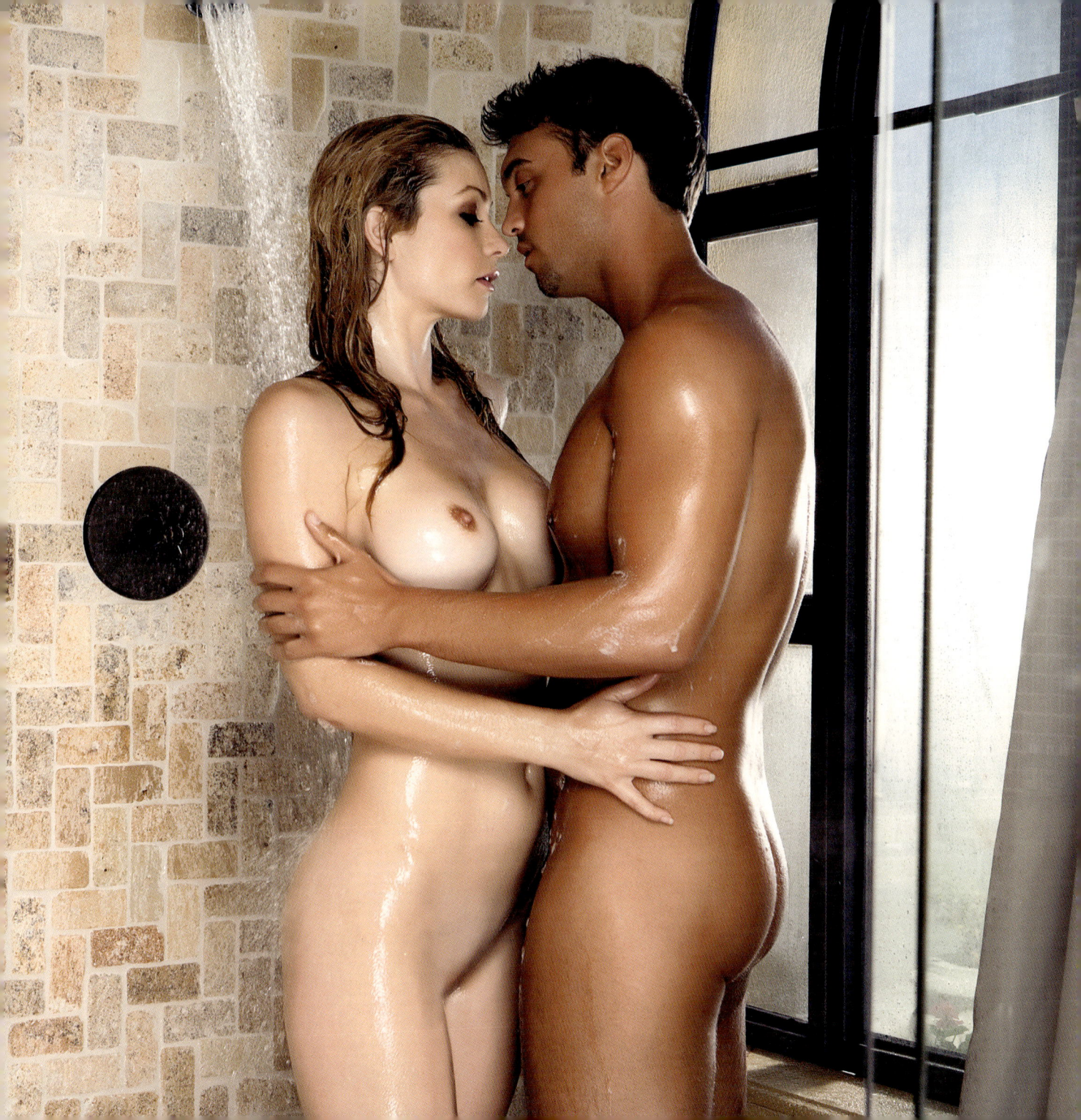

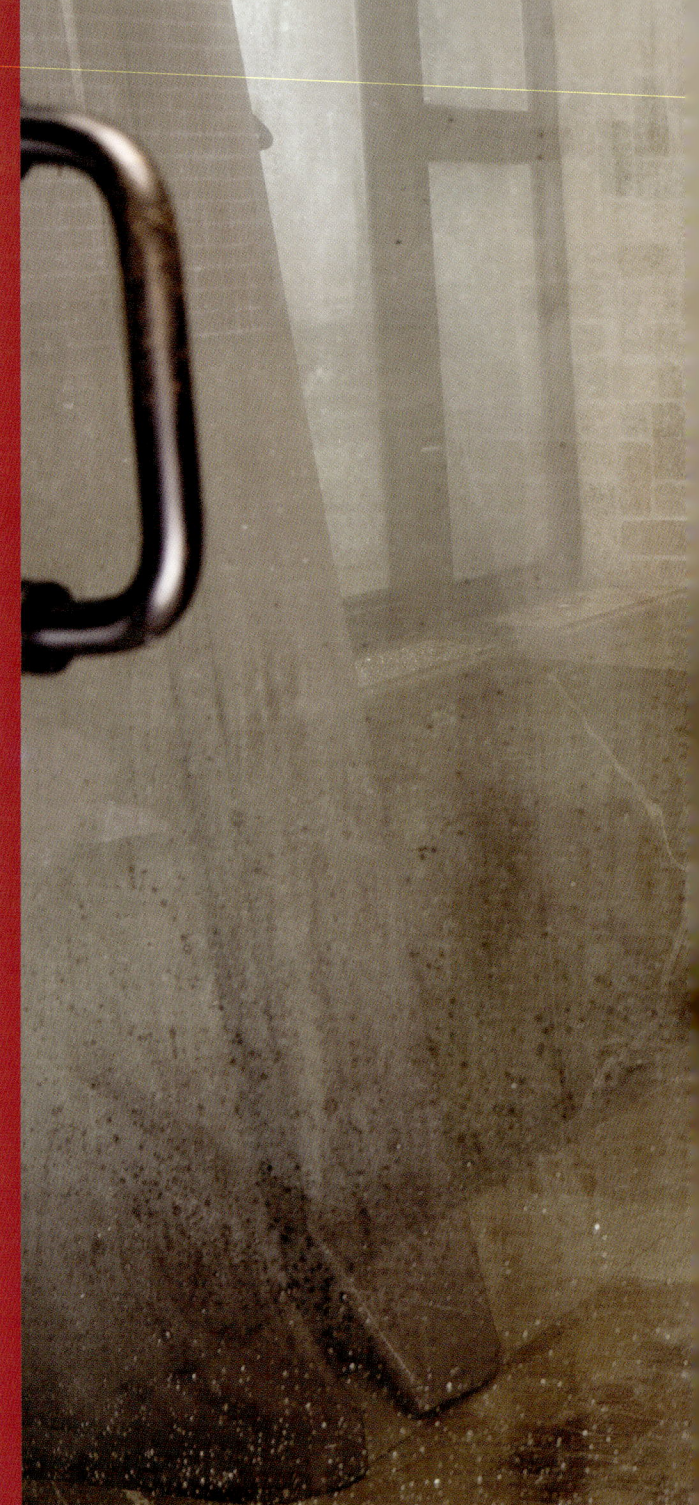

Blissful Baths

You may not have a movie star-type bathtub, but with a little preparation and a few products, the two of you can still take a bath together and enjoy every minute. One purpose of foreplay is to help you make that transition from your busy day and many worldly preoccupations into that sacred sexual space you share together. A relaxing bath can be the perfect way to leave the world behind. Here are few details to take care of before you can indulge in ideal bathing à deux.

Bathroom lighting may be great for putting on makeup or plucking your brows, but it is generally not conducive to romance. Instead of turning on those overheads, invest in some deliciously scented column candles (the fat kind, for stability), light them up, and position them around the room. If you haven't already, invest in some superthick, cushiony terry bath towels (and robes, too, if you like) large enough to envelop and warm you when you're done with the tub and ready to move the festivities elsewhere. And make sure you have some rich, emollient bath oil, preferably the bubbling kind. Bathing—especially for prolonged periods—can rob your skin of precious moisture, and a luxurious bath oil can protect you from dryness later on—plus, it makes the water feel silky. Some specific scents to look for are ylang ylang (for lust), rose (for love), and pennyroyal (for stamina).

Now you're ready to take the plunge—but this is foreplay, so have fun with it. Don't just disrobe: Do a sexy striptease for each other, using the techniques we talked about in chapter 1.

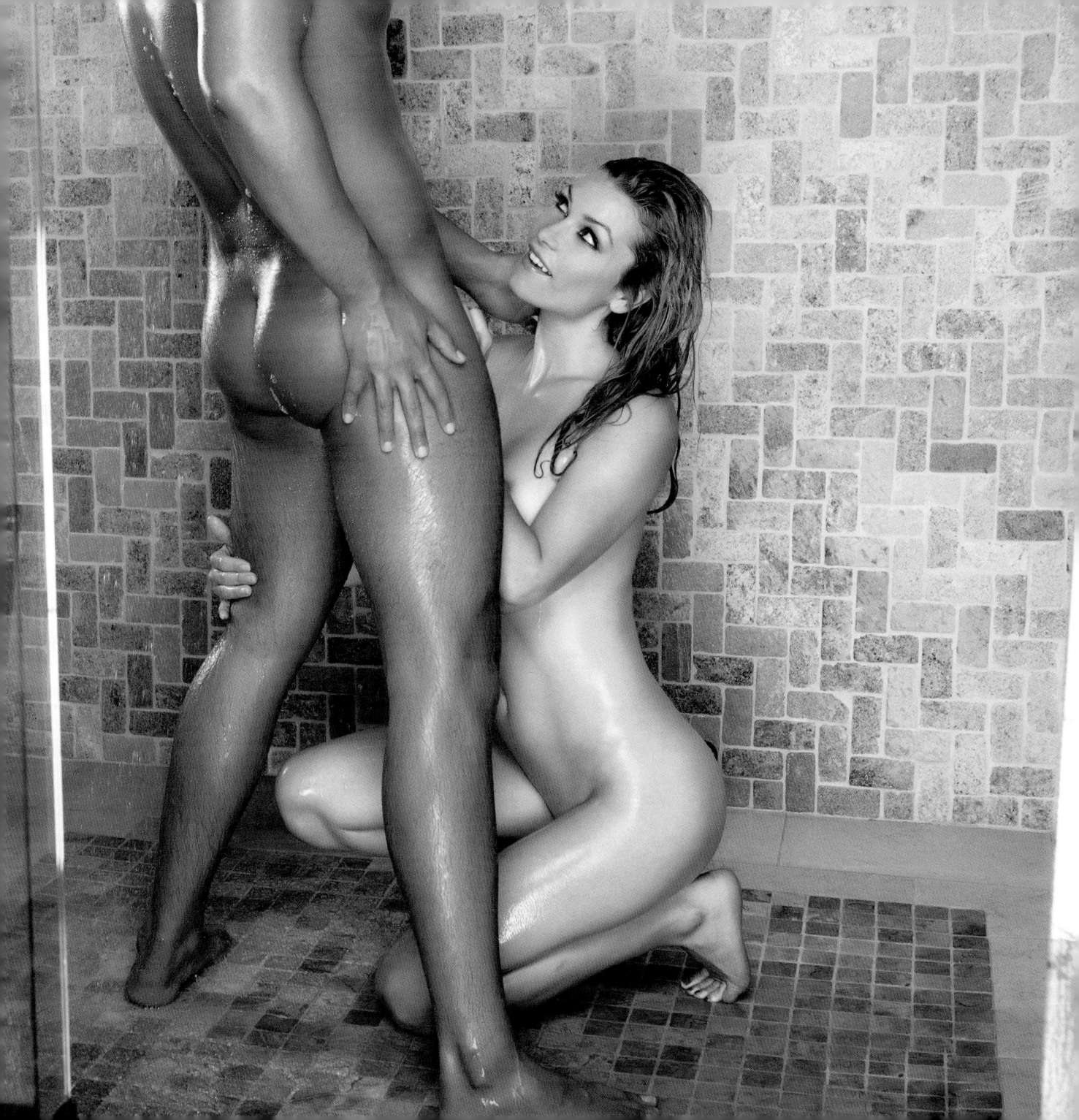

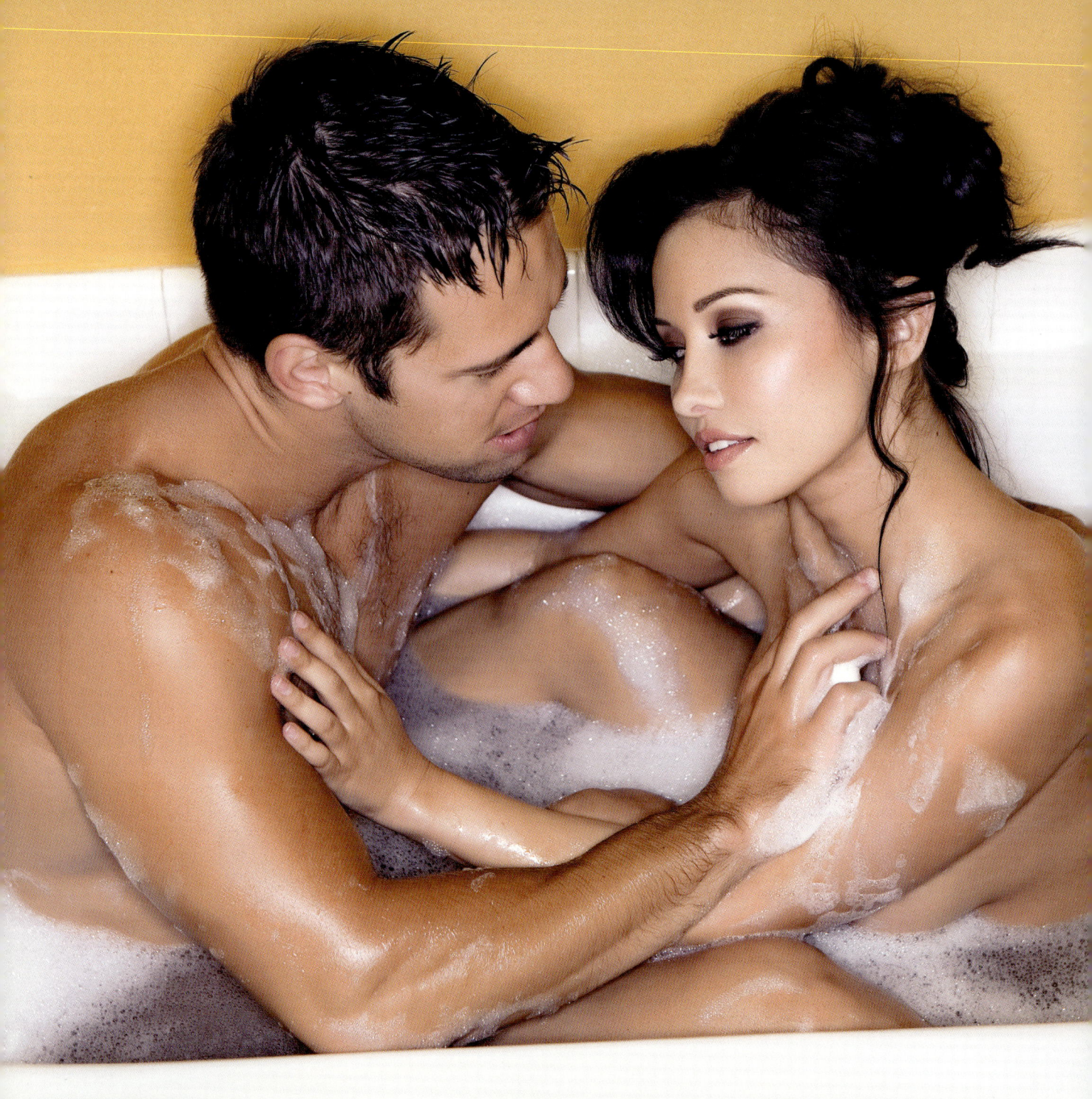

Once the bathroom is prepared, run a nice full, bubbly tubful and climb in. Make sure the water starts out a bit on the hot side because it will cool quickly. You might even want to keep the hot water trickling in as you soak, periodically lifting the stopper and letting some drain out, so that your bath retains its warmth. You want to be comfortable, so if necessary add one or more inflatable tub pillows to lean on. Now the fun begins. If you want to do more than just relax, unwind, and soak, here are a few specific ideas for bathtub fun to get you started:

Soap It Up. You lather yourself up all the time, but it's not every day that you have a sexy, eager helper. Take turns smoothing soap all over each other, paying extra special attention to the breasts (see those nipples come to attention?), buttocks, inner thighs, and other favorite erogenous zones. Do your work sensually and methodically, but take care when it comes to penetrating touch, as the water and soap can irritate sensitive vaginal and anal tissues. Soap is a lovely lubricant. Smooth it down those long, tired legs, run it over the neck, squish it between each toe . . . and when one of you has had enough, switch roles. End by sinking down into the water for a lovely rinse.

Get Grabby. Ladies, this is your opportunity to give your man's cock some serious personal attention. Soap up your hands and give him a fabulous hand-over-hand cock massage: Grasp the top of the shaft with one hand and stroke downward firmly, ending by cupping the tip just as your other hand is beginning the next stroke. Start slowly and increase the speed, hand over hand, until he's in ecstasy.

The Tongues Have It. While your lower bodies soak, let your mouths explore each other up top using all of the luscious techniques discussed in chapter 2. Kiss and suck each other all over, gradually working your way down. And if you enjoy a little underwater exploration, dive in and use those mouths underwater to tease and tantalize one another's genitals. Try blowing some bubbles down there to vibrate and stimulate your mate. By the time you come up for air, your lover will be gasping, too.

Hooking Up. Sit face to face with your legs wrapped around each other's waists, so that your pelvises are pressed together. Now use your soapy hands to explore each other's backsides, buttocks, and beautiful butt cracks to your heart's delight, running your fingers down past the anus, cupping the buttocks from below, and finally exploring every inch of each other's sexual creases and centers as your chests and abdomens remain touching. It doesn't get any closer—or hotter—than this.

Spoons. Sit one behind the other. Guys, you take the rear position first and seat your lady between your legs, right up against your cock. Now wrap your arms around her, fondle her beautiful breasts, stroke her waist, and reach down to pleasure her gently (without letting the soapy water penetrate her sensitive vagina), stroking the hood over her clitoris ever so softly. Use your hands or a washcloth to stroke her neck, shoulders, arms, and back. Ladies, lie back and enjoy the attention, turning your head to nibble his neck, ear, and cheek—then switch it up and take your turn behind.

Paint Party. The bathroom is the perfect place to get messy, so break out the nontoxic body paints (you can find them at any sex shop, or you can even use kids' fingerpaints) and go to town on each other. Paint circles and spirals around the breasts and cock, draw hearts and flowers over each other's abdomens and backs, paint a bikini on your lover, doodle polka dots on his testicles, or draw a target on her tummy and then stick your tongue in the center of it. Let your inner Van Gogh have free rein—then jump in the tub, sponge each other off, and start all over if you want.

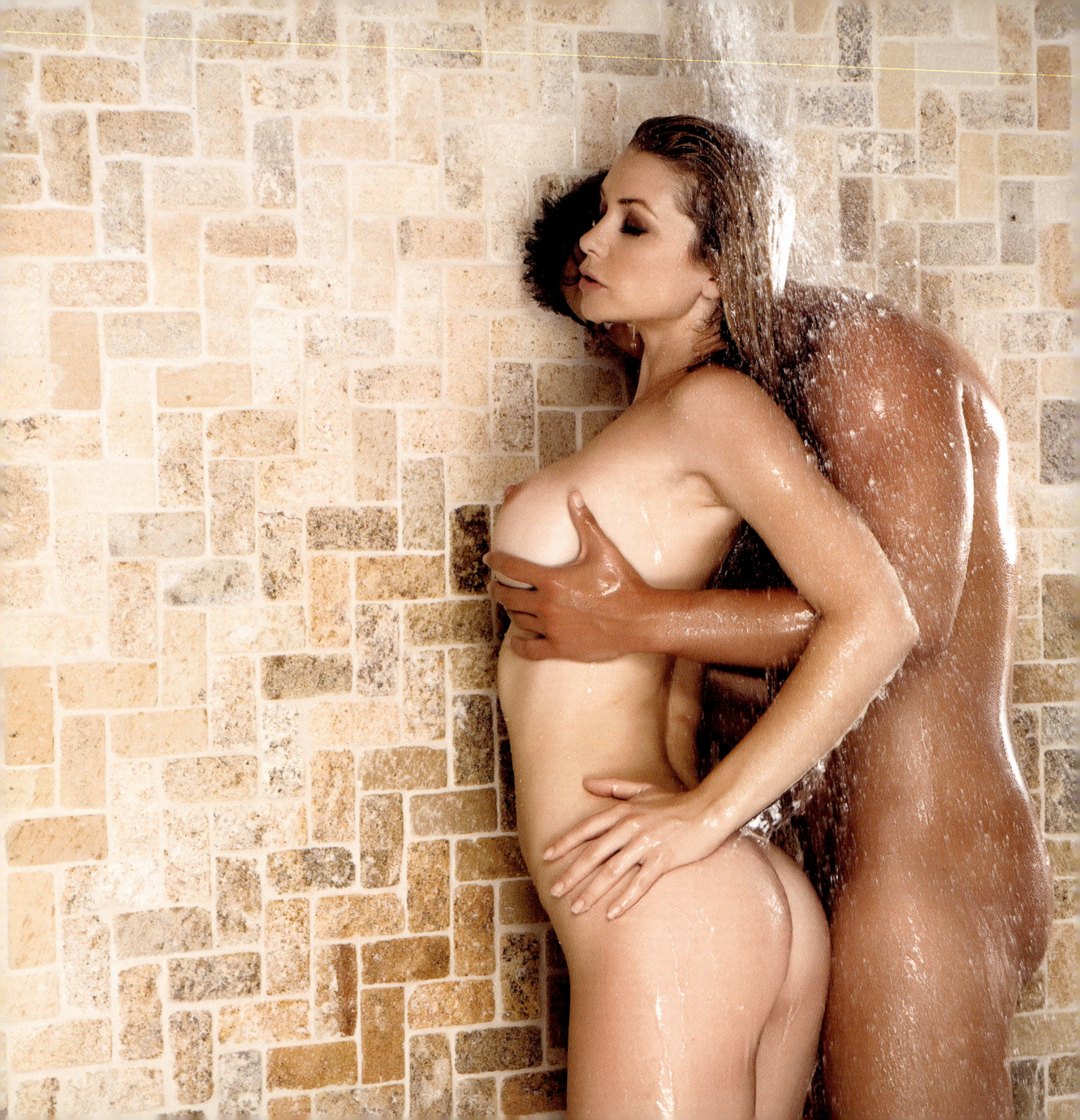

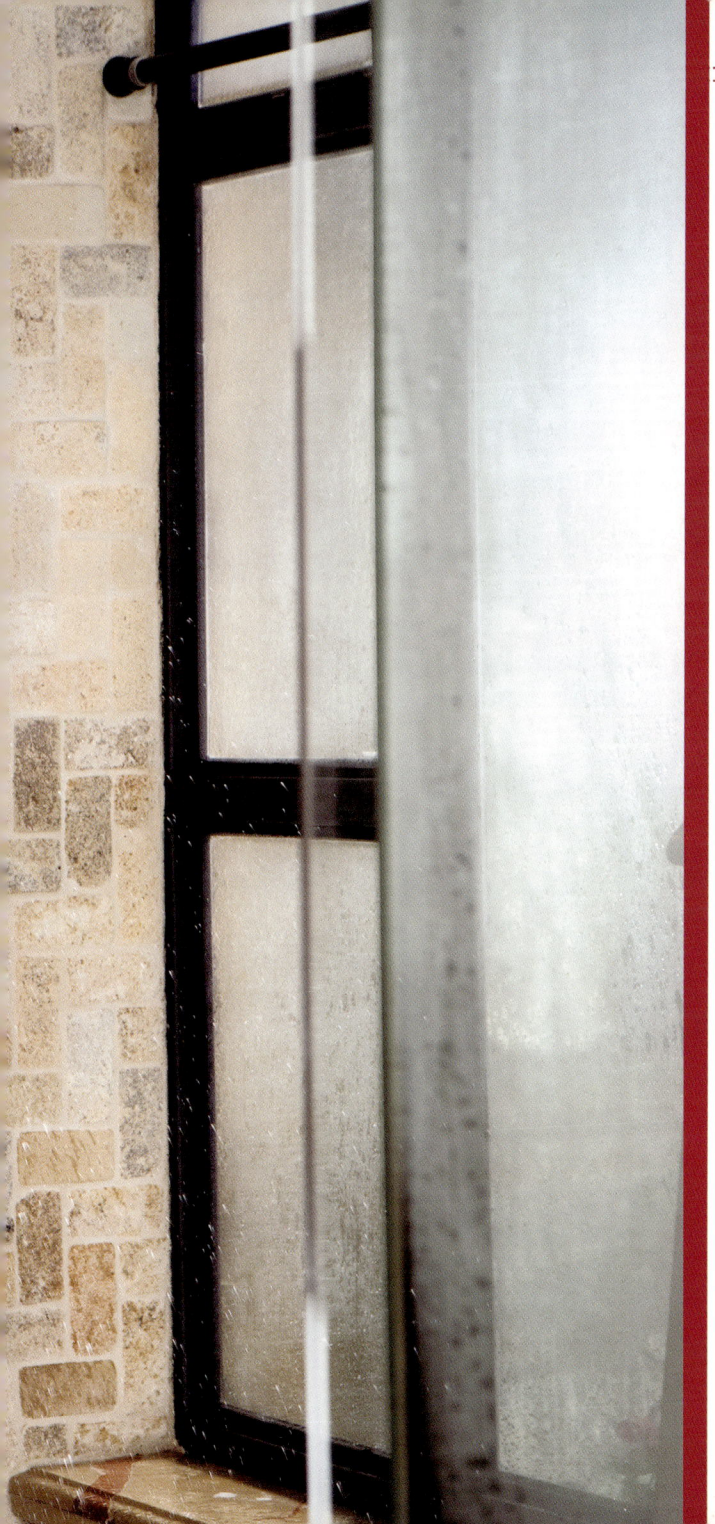

Sharing a Shower

Showers can be as sexy as baths, though perhaps a bit less relaxing and more stimulating. (A change of pace from your usual bathing routine is nice, so if you are accustomed to taking baths, try a shower together and vice versa.) Prepare the bathroom as described earlier, but make sure the bath oil you choose is suitable as shower gel, too. If you are serious about joint showers, you might want to invest in one of the many massaging showerheads on the market, which allow you to control the force, direction, and pulsation of the water. Another great option is a showerhead that you can release from the wall and use by hand (common in Europe), directing the water exactly where you want it. Select a water temperature that suits you both and climb in. Washing each other can be one of the most sensual forms of foreplay; you're sure to feel pampered, clean, cared for, and super sexy. Here are some specific tips for turning your double shower into dirty, clean fun:

Soaparific. Take turns soaping each other up, massaging the lather in from head to toe, and rinsing each other off, taking lots of time for each step. Or try simultaneous lathering, mirroring each other's techniques. You can wash each other's hair, too, providing a great excuse for a delicious head massage.

Back-Up Plan. Direct some hot water against the shower wall to warm up the tile, then back your lover against the wall, using a bit of force to show him you mean business. Then get your mouth and tongue into the action, starting with a deep, sensual kiss on his mouth and working your way down his body as the water streams over you, kissing, nipping, and lapping all the way. When you reach the promised land, take his cock in one hand while giving it a few long licks, circling the tip with your tongue and employing your favorite oral techniques from chapter 4. Give him a soaking-wet preview of the fun to come once you dry him off and get down to business.

Lady's Day. Guys, instruct your lover to stand under the water, facing the wall, and encircle her with your arms from behind. Caress her breasts, tweak her nipples, and let your hands play over her abdomen and thighs, finally exploring her mound, stroking her labia, and gently rolling her clitoris between your thumb and forefinger. Then work your mouth down her back, tonguing her spine vertebra by vertebra until you reach the crack of her ass. Explore that clean wet asshole with your tongue until she cries for mercy.

Let It Rain. Stand face to face under the most powerful stream you can handle, snug together, kissing deeply. Hold on tight to each other's buttocks. Ladies, carefully jump up and wrap your legs around your man's waist so that he is holding you, his cock pressing tight against your slit. Guys, hold on tight, cradling your lover while you probe her mouth, ears, and neck with your tongue. (Make sure you are rinsed off, so you aren't too slippery for this one.)

Working the Whirlpool

If you are fortunate enough to have access to a private hot tub or whirlpool, you're in luck. I don't think I need to elaborate on how wonderfully sensual all of that warm, powerful, swirling water can be, especially when you are sharing it. One caveat about hot tub bathing, or even the regular kind: Although a glass of champagne can be a nice accompaniment, be careful about consuming alcohol while in a tub. The combination of the damp heat and the alcohol can cause a precipitous drop in blood pressure, which can make you feel faint, especially when you stand up. There's nothing sexy about a dangerous fall or a trip to the emergency room! Whether or not you've been drinking, if you start to feel faint while submerged in the water, raise your body up so that your heart is above the water line.

That said, here are a few ideas for enhancing your hot tub experience:

Footsie. Position yourselves so that you each have a water jet at your back and give one another sensual, simultaneous foot massages, gradually working your way up the legs and calves—and as far up as you can reach.

Wraparound. Wrap your arms and legs around each other and allow the bubbling water to envelop you up to your necks. Move as if you were one person, bobbing gently, entwined as tightly as possible, kissing deeply.

Face Out. Try facing away from each other and toward the jets so that the water is pounding against your sex organs and acting as a stimulating vibrator. Then turn toward each other so that the jets stimulate your buttocks and anus, while you take over the stimulation of your own genitals. Watch each other's faces and show off for each other as you masturbate.

Orders Are Orders. Take turns directing each other: Gentlemen, instruct your lover to direct the water jet toward her anus while she plays with her clitoris or fondles her nipples as they float in the foamy water. Ladies, tell your man to place himself so that the jets are tickling and tantalizing his balls. Your lover's wish is your command.

Adult Swim

A nighttime dip in a pool, lake, or ocean can be a lovely way to transition to a night of lovemaking—especially if you are in a place where you can risk a skinny-dip! Though the water may feel cold at first, plunge right in and you are sure to warm each other up soon enough. There's nothing more liberating than being nude under the night sky. Even if you aren't a nudist by nature, the occasional swim au naturel will make you feel at one with nature, and with each other. Here are some moves for your skinny-dip:

Cradling. Take turns lying back in each other's arms and enjoying the moon and stars.

Duck, Duck. Duck all the way under water for a watery kiss. Experiment with different ways to wrap your limbs around each other in whole-body embraces, staying under as long as you can and then shooting to the surface together. That light-headed feeling will add to your all-over sensual pleasure.

Floatation Fun. Use an inflatable float or paddleboard to enhance the fun. Take turns lying back on the floatation device while your mate fondles and kisses you from head to toe as you bob gently on the water. Or go even further and ravish your mate orally while he or she floats on the waves. Have her hang her head back over the top edge of the float so you can apply upside-down kisses while fondling her breasts and nipples. Ladies, do the same with your man, tweaking his nipples and stroking his cock.

You're Naked—and I'm Not

Naked is fabulous, right? But you don't *both* have to be naked to have fun. Sometimes it is even sexier if one of you remains clothed while the other is naughtily nude. If you want to add a hint of voyeurism or dominance/submission to the festivities, take turns playing the dominant role and ordering your lover to strip down and do your bidding. There's something about watching your naked lover that can be supremely exciting, whether you are a man or a woman. (For more on this kind of edgy fun, check out chapter 6.)

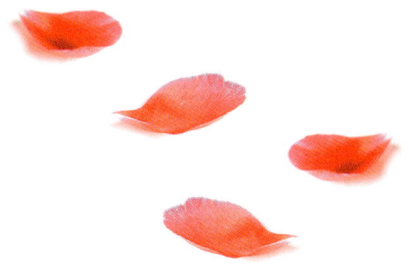

CHAPTER 8

Fun in Public

You remember the old question, "If a tree falls in the woods . . . ," right? Applying that to foreplay, the question might be, If you get the action going with nobody around to witness it, is it really a party? The answer is a resounding yes! But some of us find sex (or at least the preliminaries) doubly exciting when the canoodling is going on under people's noses.

The thrill of exposure, the proximity to other people, the under-the-table grope, or the restroom romp can be wonderful aspects of foreplay. Nothing bonds a couple better than a conspiracy of good-natured public naughtiness—and the instant gratification aspect of it will make you feel liberated and impulsive. Here are some ideas to get you started down the path of public lewdness. Final destination: bedroom fireworks!

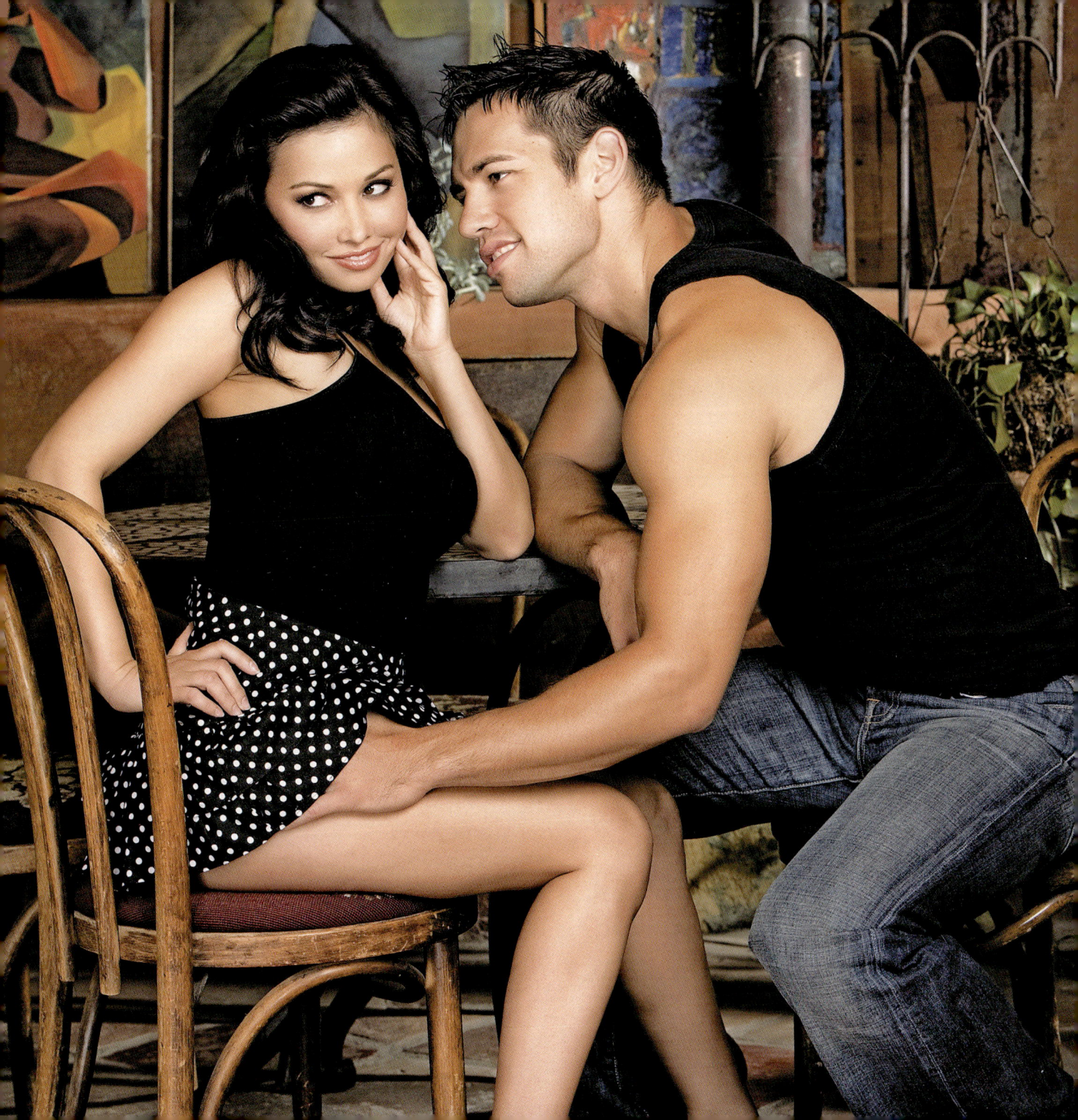

Bar None

How often have you found yourselves gazing across the table at each other during a mundane dinner or drinks date, wishing you could dispense with the polite conversation and get to the fun part of the evening? Whether you are at a table for two or out with friends, there are ways to have your cake and eat it, too—if you use a little ingenuity. Spot that gleam in your lover's eye? Call his bluff.

Footsie Fun. Ladies, this is when those slip-on (slip-OFF) pumps come in handy. Slide your foot out of your shoe and use it to let your mate know you are thinking about the wicked things you intend to do to him later. Start by exploring his ankle, sliding your tootsies as far up his pant leg as it will allow. If you are seated across from him, go ahead—place your pretty foot right against his crotch and give it a nice caress. Press and prod him with your toes until you can feel his cock start to get interested and strain against his fly. If you can manage it, undo his belt or slide his zipper down. Make sure to gaze into his eyes as you foot-fondle him . . . and give him a wink to show him that what's going on down there is your little secret! No one else at the table or in the restaurant need know that the sex games have begun.

Handyman. Guys, it's time for you to get in on this action. If you are sitting at a table with tablecloths, you can have a little camouflaged fun. Without breaking the conversation, reach over and give your girl's thigh a nice caress. If she's smart, she'll snuggle closer so you can reach between her legs and give her a nice little stroke, a tweak, or a grope. Start out over her clothes, but if you can, find a way to penetrate the layers. If she's wearing a skirt, reach right under it and stroke her silk panties until they are soaking wet with her juices, then let your fingers crawl right inside those panties and into her hot slit, where you can tweak her clit and even bring her to orgasm if the fancy strikes you. If she's wearing pants, it'll be a little trickier, but be bold. Go ahead and open her fly and plunge in, probing all the way. Don't forget to lick your fingers a little when you're done, to show her how much you love the way she tastes. If you play it carefully, nobody but the two of you will have any idea how hot this date is getting!

Taking a Powder. If the two of you are getting so turned on that you just can't wait 'til you get home, you can try to find a bit of privacy on the spot. Where you end up depends on your level of daring and the setup of the facilities. Lots of restaurants and bars have unisex, single bathrooms—in which case, help yourselves to a private room for two. (Even if the bathrooms are designated "Men" and "Women," if they are singles with doors that lock, you can share one with alacrity.)Two notes: First, be considerate—don't take too long and risk emerging to the sight of a long line of uncomfortable people. And second . . . no need to go all the way. Remember that in sex, anticipation is half the fun, so enjoy a hot "appetizer"—a little necking, a fast grope, some heavy fondling and fingering that'll have you desperately trying to stifle your moans of bliss—but save the main course for later. Readjust your clothing, reapply your makeup, and head back to the table before anyone has time to wonder where you've gone.

Other Options. Bathrooms, closets, or even garages can be turned into semiprivate trysting places, as well (though—again—if you barricade yourselves in the bathroom, make sure there's another one available for guests who've had too much beer!). Bathrooms, in general, aren't very conducive or comfortable for prolonged sex play, but the harsh lighting and cold tile can be thrilling for a few minutes of illicit fun—and they are certainly useful for freshening up afterward.

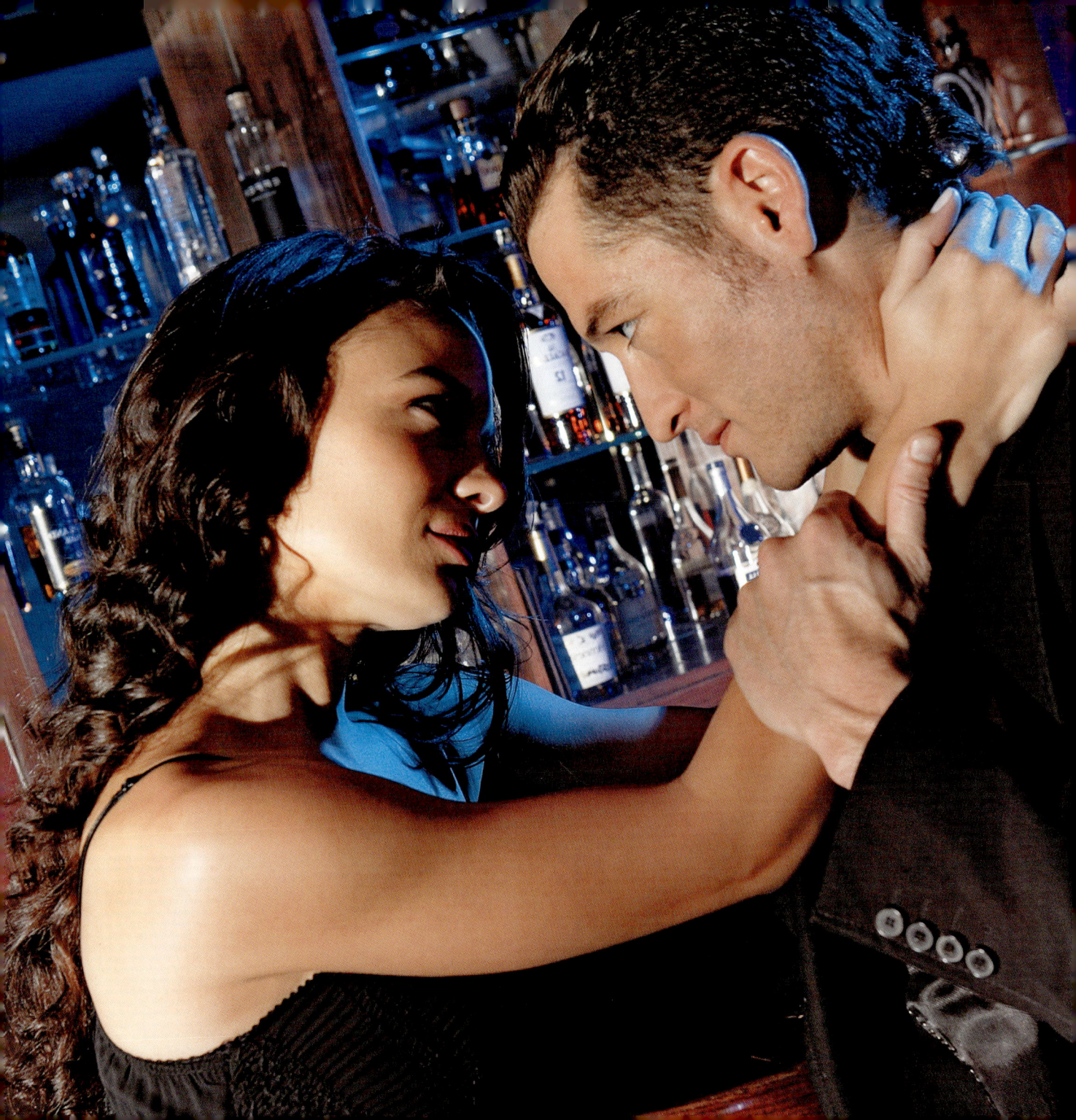

It's OUR Party

When I was a little girl, I loved when my parents had parties. I'd go into the room where all of the guests had laid their coats on the bed, climb up, and just. . .wallow in all of that fur! I didn't know it at the time, but I was having one of my first truly sensual experiences. Here are some party ideas:

Guest Room. As an adult, I still love that room! Next time you find yourselves at a party with a craving to get physical, find the coatroom (or any spare bedroom), close the door, and have a private soiree of your own. Suck and stroke each other to distraction, enjoying the thrill of knowing that someone could barge in at any moment; to enhance that thrill, leave the door unlocked but be ready to dive *under* those coats if necessary.

Party On. That quick romp at the party is a delicious preliminary to what you'll be up to when you finally make it to home sweet home. Don't let things get so hot and heavy that you run out of steam, though. We're talking foreplay here—heightened by the thrill of potential discovery and the delight of a shared secret as you wend your way back to the buffet. (You've whetted your appetite, after all!) Enjoy the hospitality of friends in whatever way you can dream up, but don't risk wearing out your welcome or your libidos.

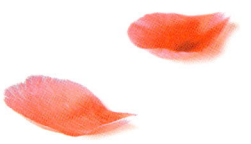

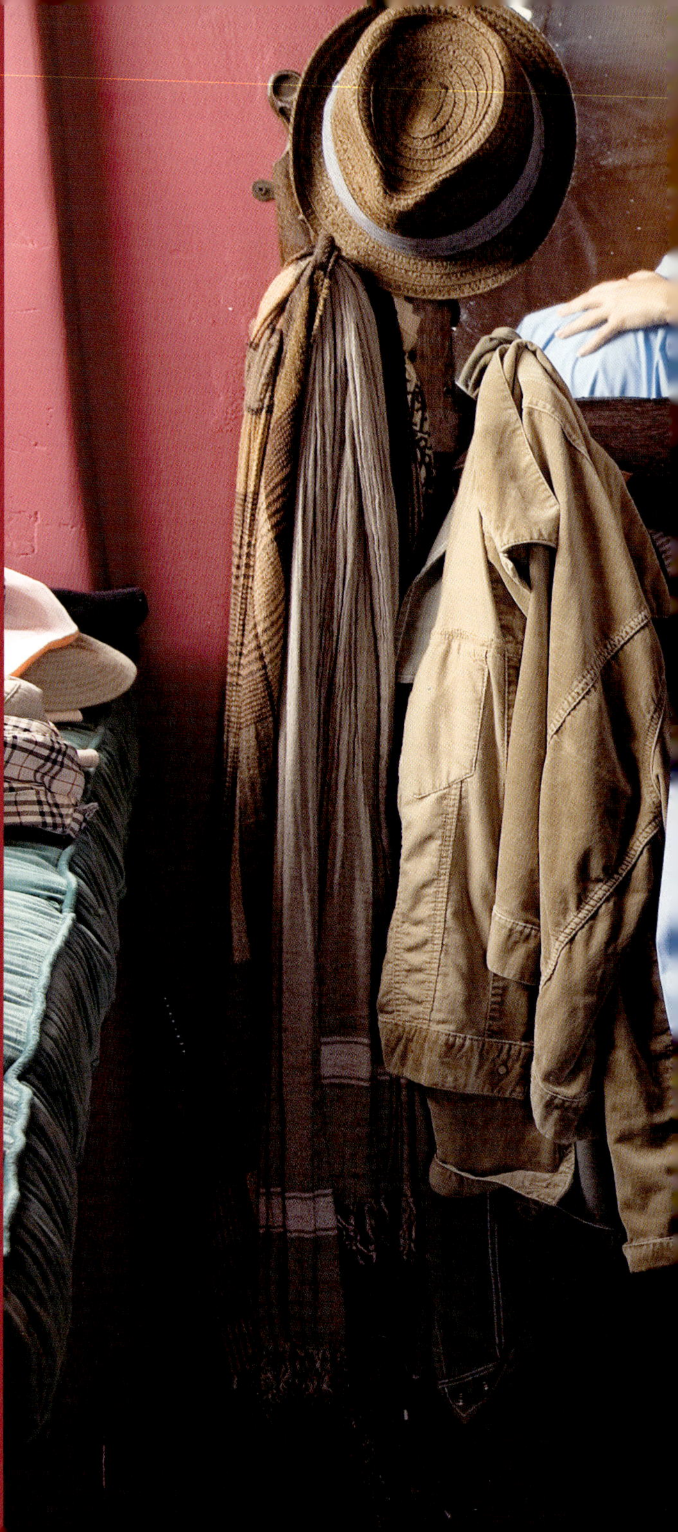

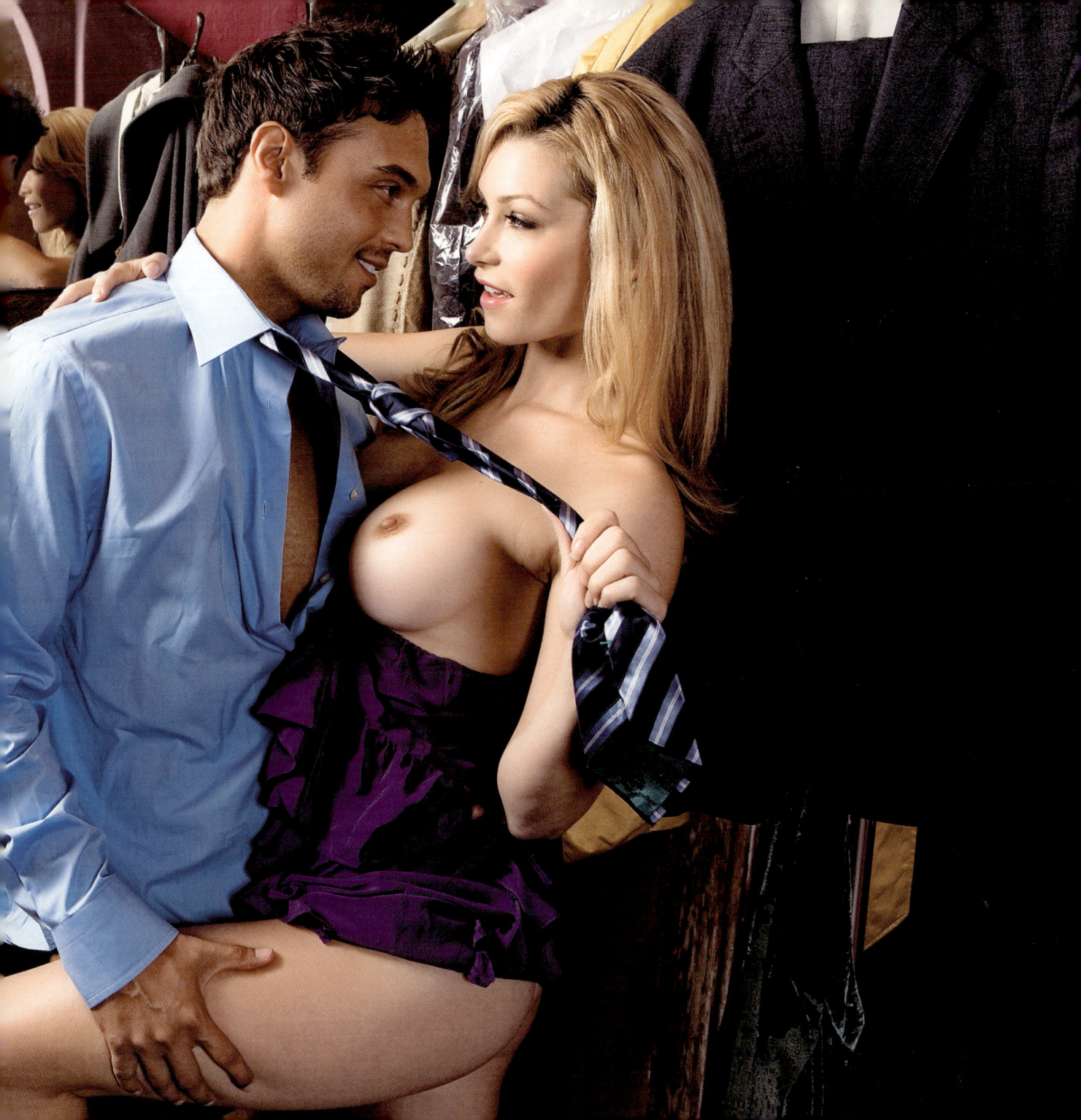

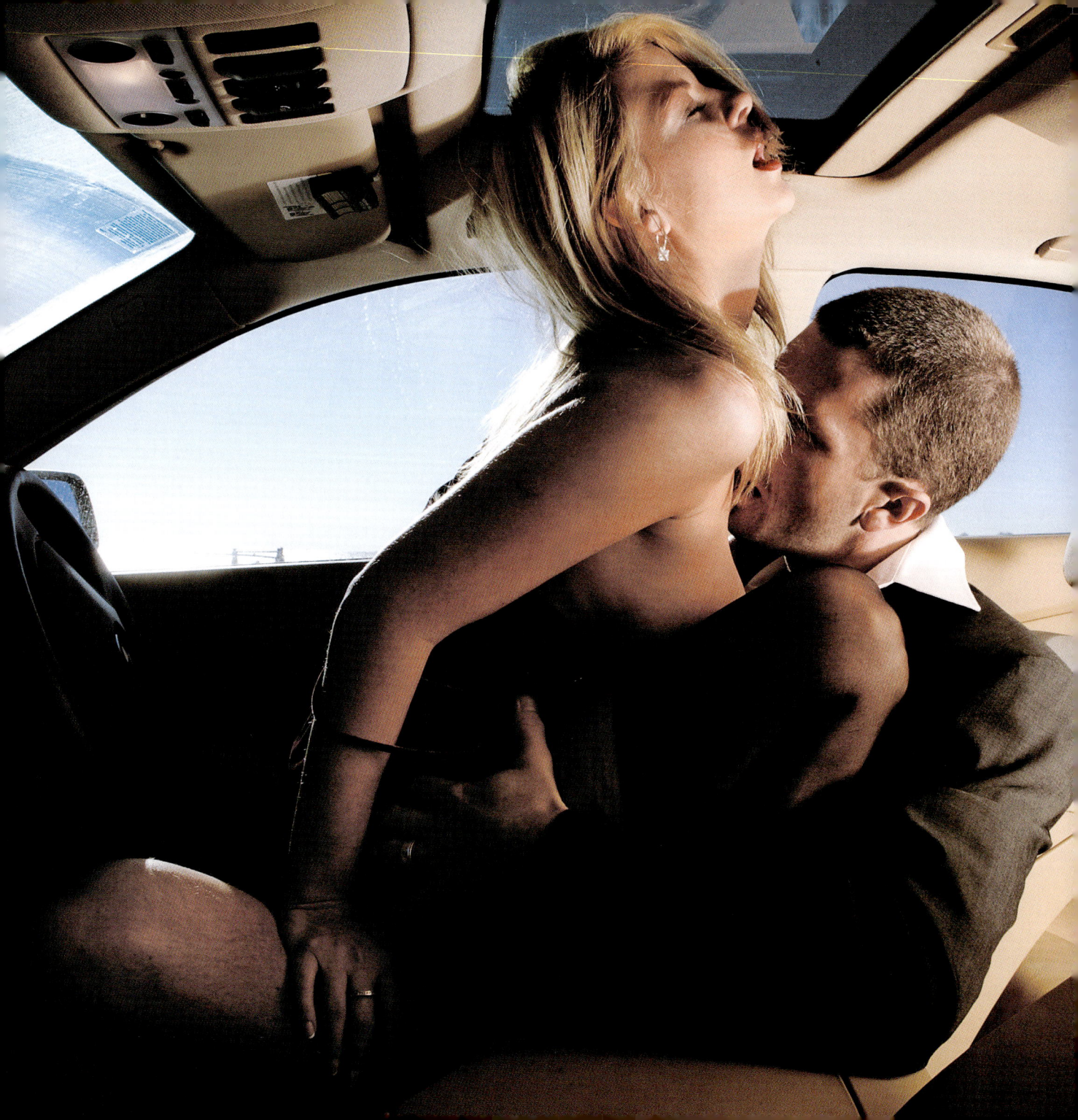

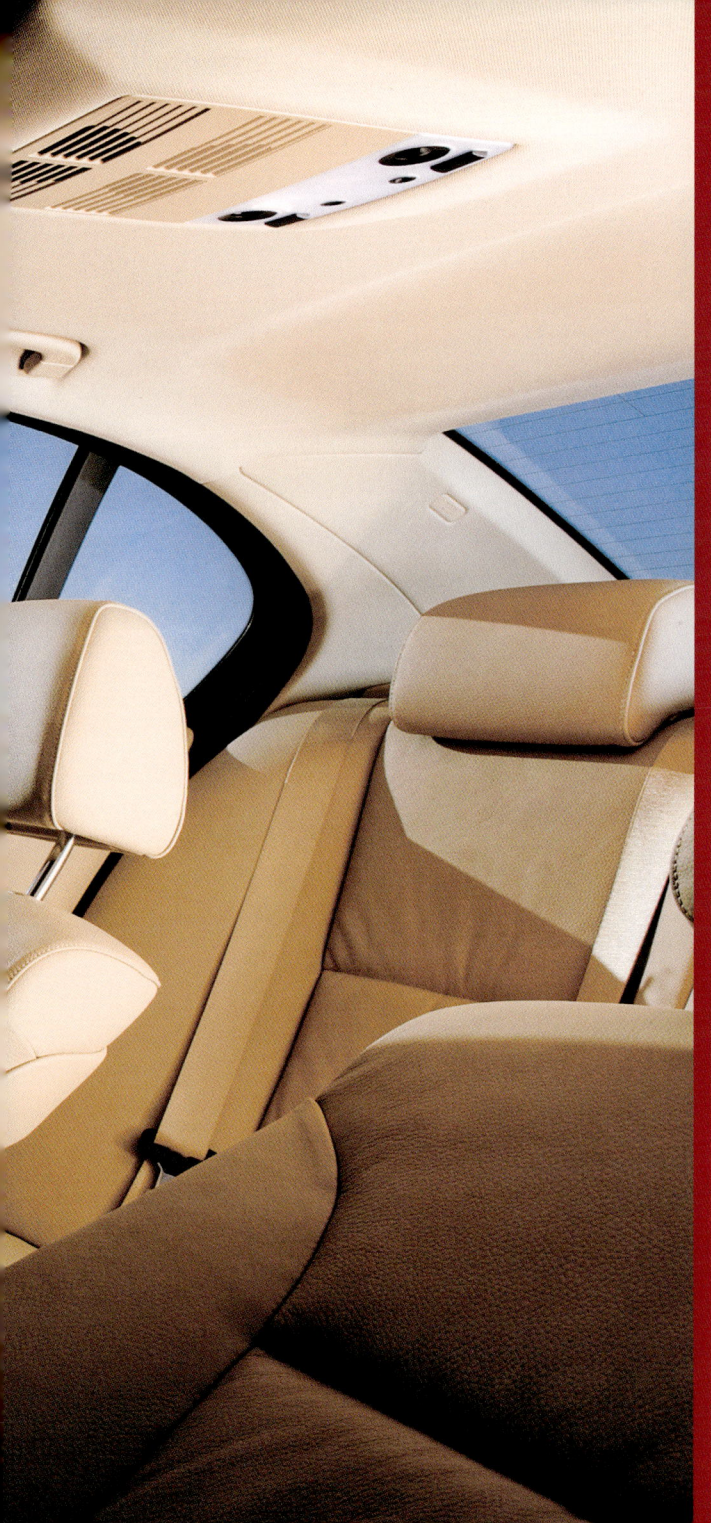

Baby, You Can Drive My Car

Autoerotic doesn't refer to sex in a car—but maybe it should! Lots of us had our first adult sexual experiences in a car, and it's still a classic venue for a furtive grope. If you haven't steamed up a windshield since high school, find an opportunity to grab your guy's gearshift for some automotive foreplay. To ensure that you don't break any traffic laws or put yourselves or others in danger, confine your car play to a parked vehicle—and leave the stunt driving to movie actors! Try these moves:

Up Front. First order of business is to find a secluded spot to park—maybe someplace with a nice view but not a lot of people around. (Or there's always the drive-in, though there aren't many of those left these days.) And hey, how convenient is it that you've got a great stereo system all set to go? Pick out a sexy CD and avoid commercials and traffic reports. Front seats tend to be divided these days, as opposed to the old bench seats from the '50s and '60s, but that shouldn't slow you down too much. Ladies, try straddling your man right in the driver's seat. If that's a bit too cozy, improvise: The space restriction is part of what makes the whole thing challenging—and hot. You'll find somewhere to put all of those limbs, and you might engineer some new moves in the process.

Backseat Driver. Of course if you're really serious about car games, the backseat is the way to go. Go ahead and relive your teenage glory days, when the car was the only private necking spot you could find. If you intend to shed any clothing, bring along a soft blanket. It'll provide a nice cushion between you and those sticky vinyl seats, and a way to cover up and keep warm, too. Ladies, dive under that blanket to suck and lick your lover's cock until he's ready to explode. Guys, turn your lady facedown on that seat and give her beautiful ass a tongue bath, penetrating right down her crack and into her anus with your tongue. But don't get so carried away that you forget to be on the lookout for police officers with 1,000-watt flashlights!

All Work—and a Little Play, Too!

Fooling around at the office? Why not! Try a few of these:

Late-Night Visit. This one comes in handy if your mate is working too hard and you feel the need to distract him. Show up after closing time, when there are few people around. Find a cushy office—not your lover's (remember, you are trying to get him *away* from all of that work)—and show him what you have on under that raincoat. Nothing? Wow! The couch, the carpet, and even that big mahogany desk make great spots for an invigorating little work break. Bend him backward over the desk and give him the blow job of his life. Make him stand with his bare cock against the office window while you rub your breasts all over his back, ass, and thighs. Seat him in the desk chair and straddle him face to face, grinding your pelvises together as you kiss and fondle each other. When you've had enough office play, pour him a nice drink from the thermos you brought and let him get back to his deadlines, promising sweet completion of what you started the minute he walks in the door.

Kissing Colleagues. If you work together *and* play together, it's bound to cross your minds. Why not get it on without leaving the office? If your relationship is a secret (some companies frown on such fraternization), use extra discretion—but where there's a will, there's a way, and there's a special thrill that comes from ripping each other's clothes open in the same conference room where you held a serious business meeting just hours earlier. What's that big table for, if not to make it your personal playground? Or better yet, slip under that table, open your zippers and buttons, and reach inside for some superhot hand jobs. If you want to prepare for your office tryst (not everything has to be totally spontaneous to be fun), pack a sexy little meal to share afterward and stash it in the office fridge. Include a bottle of wine—if you don't have to get back to work, that is.

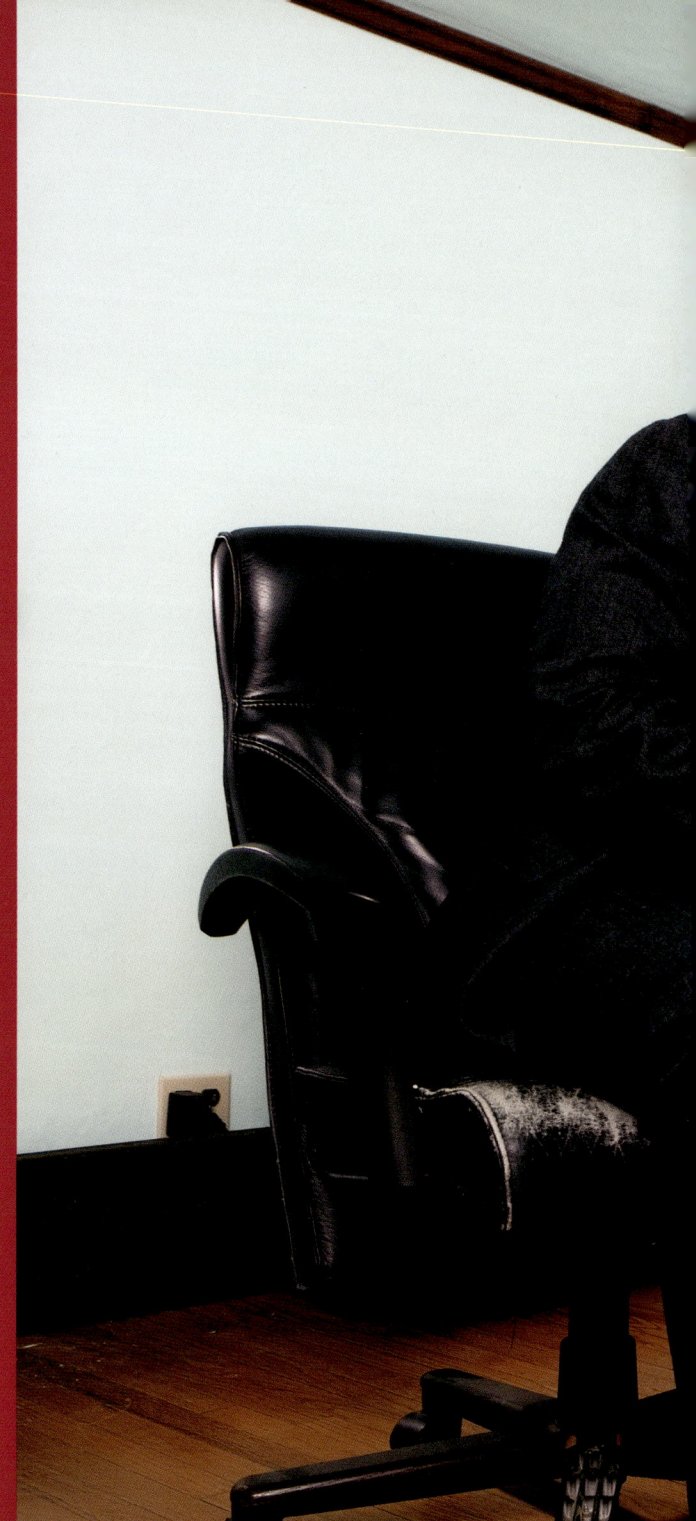

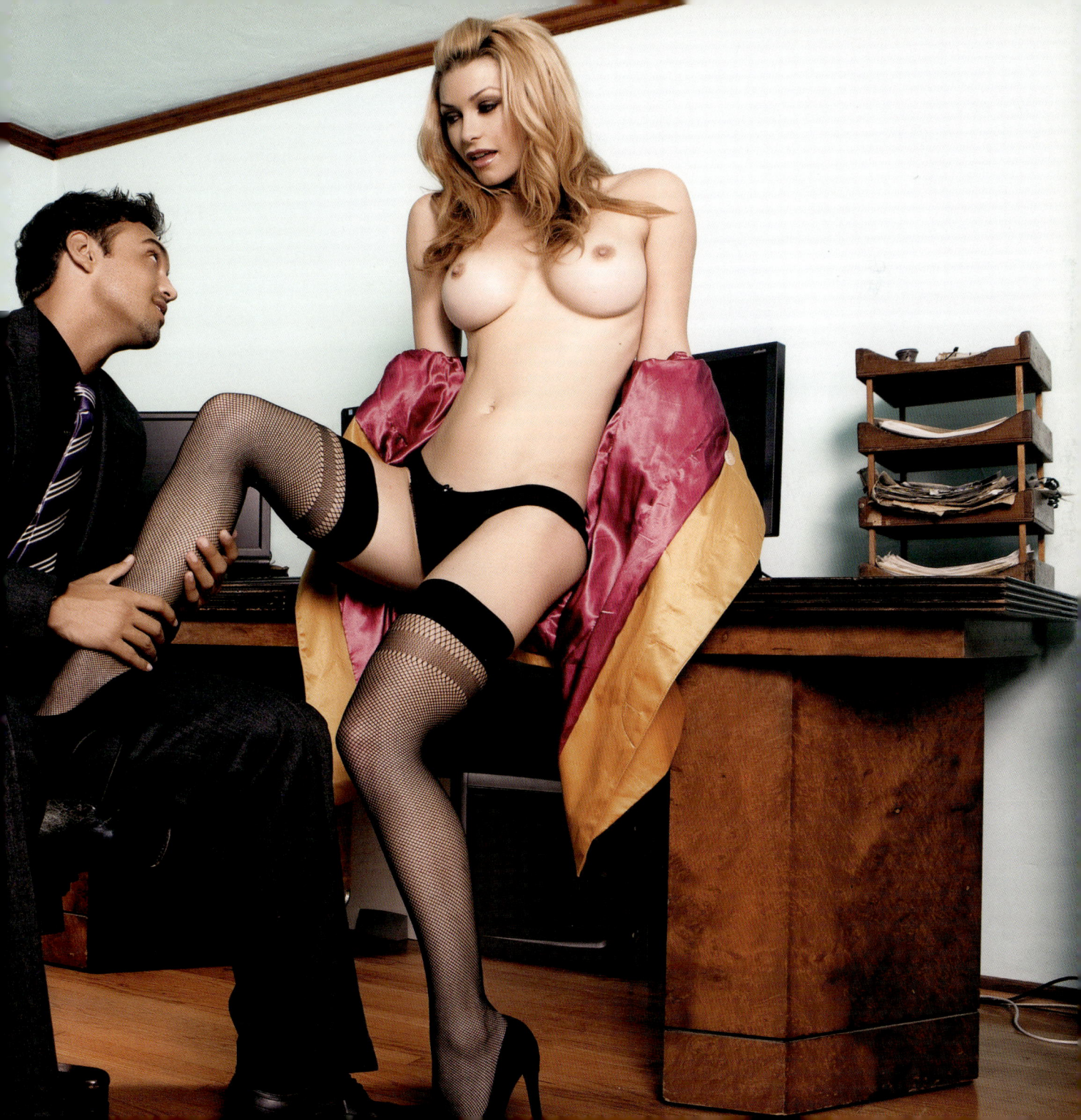

Going Down? One last tip: A quick grope in the elevator can be wicked and really fun. Don't pull the emergency switch—you don't want that alarm to go off—but, depending on how long it takes you to go from your office to the lobby, there might be time to grab his crotch and give it a squeeze, plant a luscious kiss on his lips, and grab his sweet behind with both hands as you slip your tongue down in his mouth. By the time you reach the lobby, he might need to hold his briefcase in front of him on his way to the bus!

The Great Outdoors

There's nothing like open-air horseplay . . . nothing. Just use a little creativity and the wide-open sky is the limit:

Beach Blanket Bingo. How much explanation do you need? If you can find a secluded stretch of beach (dusk is a lovely time, or even after dark, if you won't be breaking any local ordinances), you can enjoy some sexy fun under the sky, including erotic massages and delicious outdoor oral. Don't forget the sunscreen, and resign yourselves to a bit of sand in the ointment, as it were. If you feel like reenacting the love scene from *From Here to Eternity*, you won't be the first. For more on water, see chapter 7.

Life's a Picnic. Food, wine, the outdoors, and each other. Turn a wholesome "Andy of Mayberry" afternoon into an adult experience by making dessert of each other after the feast has been cleared away. Public parks and nature preserves provide lots of secluded spots, but beware of birdwatchers with big binoculars.

Rounding the Bases. If you and your lover enjoy live sports, consider a little private halftime show or seventh-inning stretch during your next home game. What happens under the stadium blanket *stays* under the stadium blanket—so bring a nice big one, draw it up to your chins, and let your hands roam inside one another's clothing, and even inside *each other*, if it strikes your fancy.

In the Air and On the Ground

Yes, Virginia, there is a Mile-High Club—but you don't have to join it in order to have a little fun in flight. (Full-on sex in an airplane bathroom would probably be considered a security breach nowadays, anyway.) And talking about hotel sex in the "in public" chapter may not seem logical, but it will when you think about it. Check these tips out:

Just Plane Fun. Like I said, this isn't about squeezing yourselves into that tiny lavatory for some acrobatic sex—though, if that's your thing, go for it. But there you are, side-by-side in your recliners for a few hours with nothing to do but watch a lousy movie. Put those complimentary blankets to good use and have some discreet fun letting your hands grope, stroke, and fondle each other. If you are on an overnight flight where they dim the lights so everyone can nap, all the better. A steamy make-out session will help pass the time. (Didn't you ever wonder why those center armrests are moveable?)

Do Not Disturb. Hotel sex can be great dirty fun—but if you think of it as private, think again. Haven't you ever settled in to your king-size hotel bed only to overhear a vigorous session unfolding in the next room or upstairs? Even luxurious hotels tend to have thin walls, so you can assume your performance may have an audience. That's especially true at motels and bed-and-breakfasts, where you have the added attraction of sharing breakfast with your "listeners" the next morning. (Smirk.) If you get off on the idea of having listeners, fooling around in a hotel, motel, inn, or guesthouse can be an exciting change of pace. Plus, you won't have to make the bed!

Now do you get the picture? Foreplay isn't just about technique, it's about scenery, changing it up, raising the bar, keeping each other guessing—and sometimes, it's about asking for a little trouble!

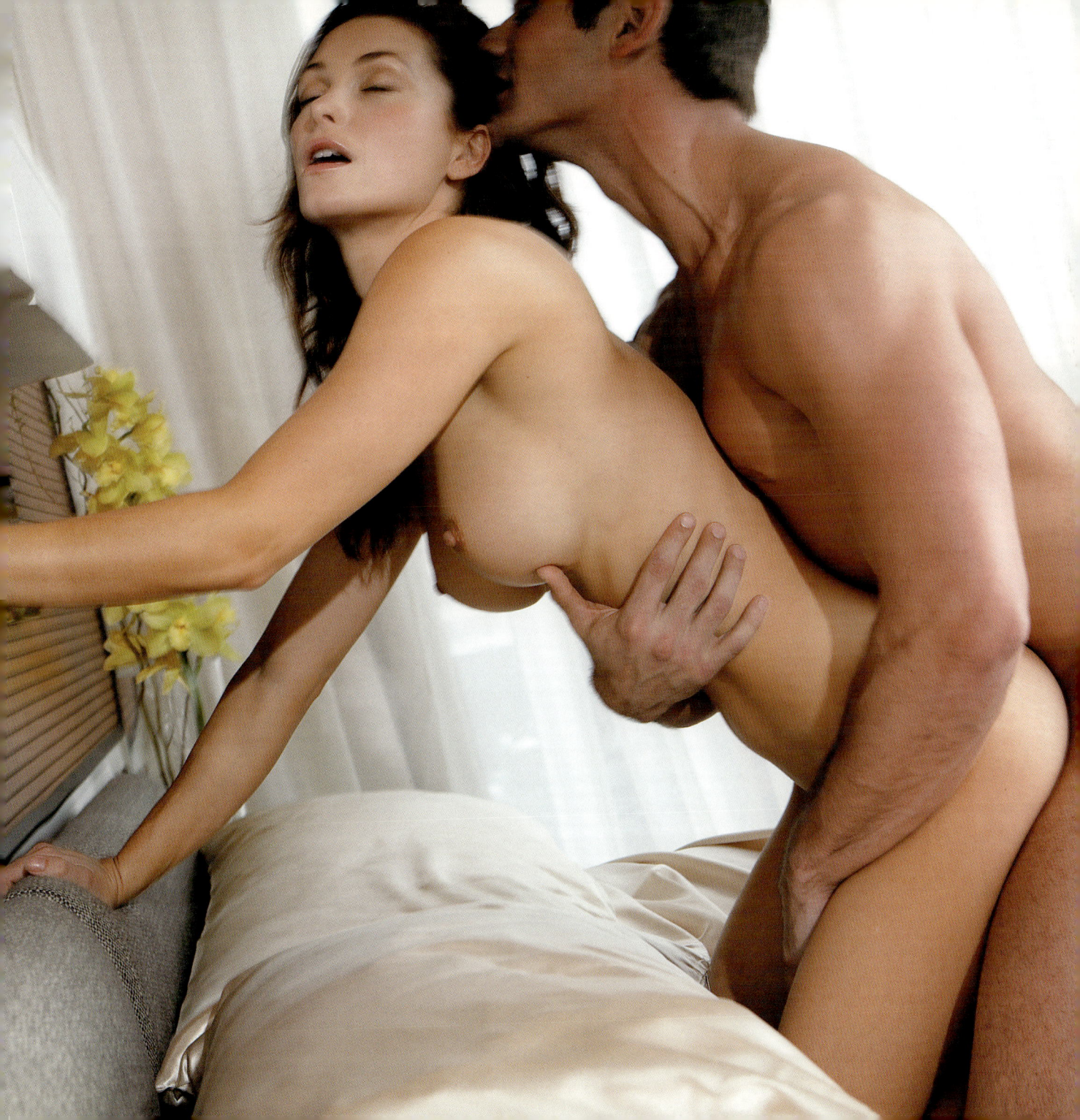

The *Other* Oral Sex: Talking!

CHAPTER 9

Throughout our foreplay journey together, I've often touched upon the importance of good communication between partners as a means to a mind-blowing sex life. Every aspect of foreplay is a kind of communication, of course, but when you get down to it, talking is the most direct form we've got. It's hard to deny that free-flowing, verbalized fantasies and well-timed, well-articulated instructions make us all better, uninhibited, confident, and intimately connected lovers. I'm not suggesting that you talk each other to death rather than getting down to the business of pleasure; I'm simply telling you that learning to open up verbally as well as physically is key. But when it comes to talking, what time is the right time?

There are two answers to that question, so I've divided this chapter into two sections. One deals with talking *about* sex—something we can all learn to be better at—and the other with talking *during* sex (and during foreplay, too), an important addition to any happy couple's sensual repertoire.

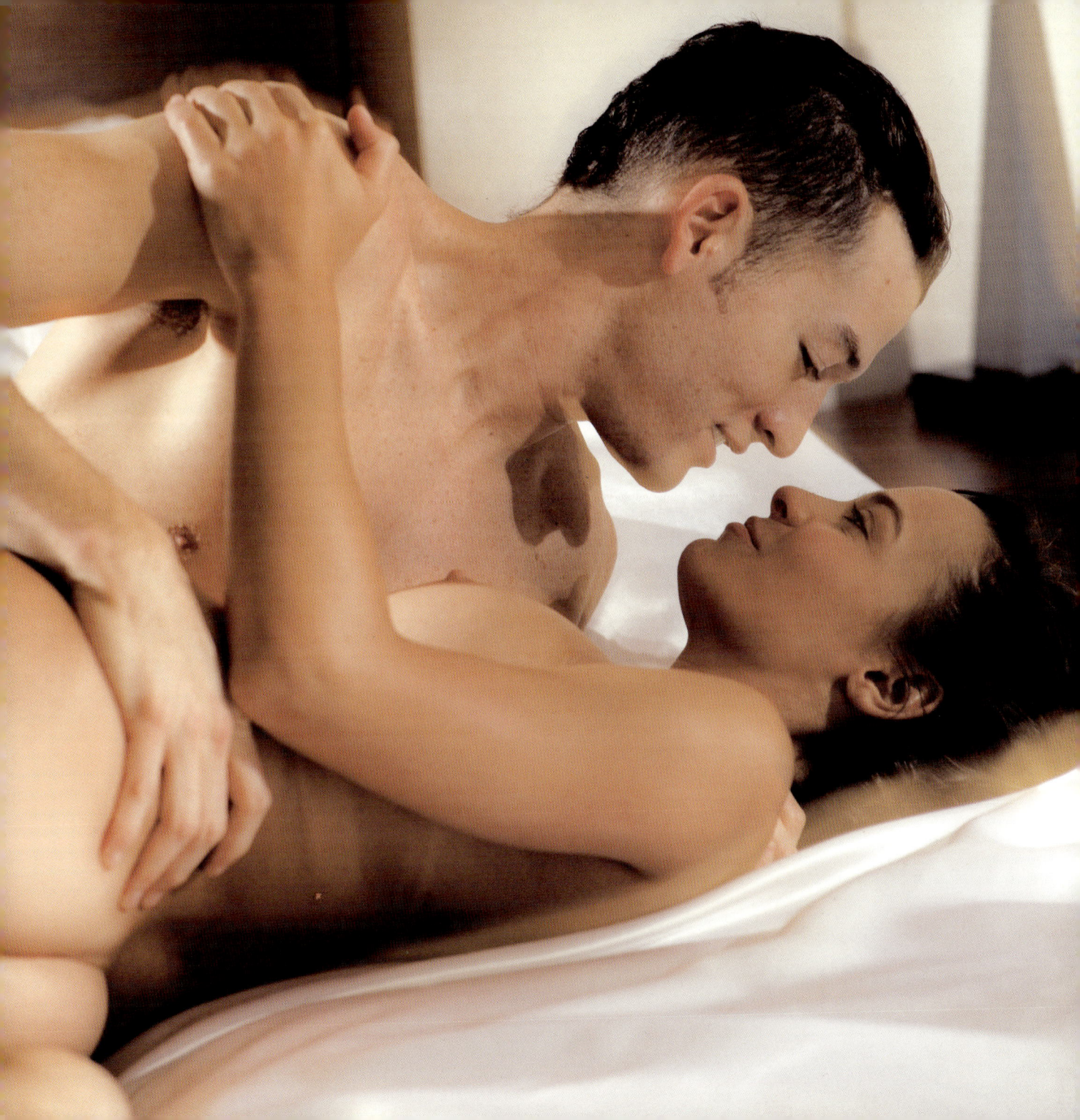

Let's Talk About It

You may not consider a heart-to-heart talk about what goes on in the bedroom part of foreplay, per se, but it can certainly enhance all that follows. You may not even feel comfortable talking on the topic at *all*—but I hope I can convince you to move past that discomfort and open up a frank dialogue about love and sex (especially sex!) with your mate. It might be the first conversation of many, and it is sure to lead to sweeter satisfaction for both of you.

Here's the main thing to remember: Everyone wants to know more about sex, about giving and receiving pleasure. And your partner would surely love to know more about what makes you weak in the knees. Is there something you'd like him to do that he hasn't gotten around to yet? There are ways to clue him in without dampening his spirits (or causing his erection to wane). Do you wonder if she is enjoying that special move you invented? You don't have to read her mind to find out. And what about that new area of sex play or position you've been dying to try? Perhaps your lover has been fantasizing about it as well. Time to compare notes!

Venturing into the wilds of sexual experience together means teaching each other what you know and feel, learning from each other gladly, and, ultimately, soaring into the stratosphere of mutual satisfaction. It all starts with a few well-chosen words:

When and Where. You want to talk to your lover about sex, but what's the right time to bring it up? There are lots of answers to that one, but the better question is, what's the *wrong* time? Answer: in the heat of the moment. Don't get me wrong—talking during sex is great fun and a big turn-on, and I'll go into that in a minute; but if you want to talk *about* sex, it's best to open that can of worms elsewhere. Let's say you'd like to explore your mate's feelings about anal sex or bondage games. Or you're wondering whether your oral sex technique is all he wants it to be. Or whatever. Whether you want to bring up a problem, open a new door, or ask for some feedback, choose a neutral–nurturing–time and place to do it in. Most important, make sure you both have time to have a relaxed conversation. (Don't start the dialogue just as she is running off to an important meeting or her favorite TV show is about to begin.) Second, choose a place where you have privacy and feel comfortable—not a noisy restaurant or crowded subway platform. Home is usually best, over a meal (the addition of a cocktail isn't a bad idea—unless it's breakfast, of course), on the couch, or hanging out in the backyard. Or take a leisurely walk around the neighborhood, hold hands, and open your hearts. Any conversation—but especially a sensitive or intimate conversation—is easier if it takes place in a relaxed and inviting setting.

How. The tone and spirit of your talk is as important as choosing a time and place, of course, so spend a little time thinking about how to approach your lover with what is on your mind. Here are my five basic rules to help you get the ball rolling:

1. **Start by saying something positive—and keep those encouraging words coming throughout the conversation, too.** "I loved it so much last night when you [*fill in the blank*]" or "Your cock is so delicious, I dream about tasting it." Be honest, of course, but focus on what's great before moving on to any problems you might want to bring up.

2. **Get to the point.** Preliminaries are fine, but don't beat around the bush *too* long. There's no reason to leave your (slightly nervous) lover hanging. "Here's what I'm wondering: Have you ever thought about trying a little [*whatever*]?"

3. **Be specific, never vague or general.** Whether your issue is the frequency of your lovemaking or a specific act you'd like to try, put your cards on the table without shame or apology. Remember, this is your lover you are talking to. No need to fear.

4. **Make it a dialogue, not a speech.** Pause frequently so your lover can ask a question or add a comment, and if the conversation starts to get a little heated or defensive, work to keep the tone calm and positive. You don't want your constructive talk to escalate into an argument. And perhaps most important . . .

5. **Don't pass judgment.** The purpose of talking about sex is to draw you closer together as a couple, not drive a wedge between you. If you need a few helpful examples of how best to talk the talk and come out stronger on the other side, read on!

What. What exactly is on your mind? Here are some of the basic kinds of topics you might want to discuss with your lover. Don't worry: You're not strange or alone. When groups convene to talk frankly about their issues concerning sex, these are the things that crop up most frequently:

1. **Foreplay—or the lack thereof.** One way to say this: "I need more preparation for the big event." (Keep this book handy for this conversation!)

2. **Sameness.** "Our lovemaking has gotten routine; there aren't enough surprises. What can we do to spice things up a little bit?"

3. **What I like.** "I love it when you do *that*, but this other thing isn't right for me."

4. **What you like.** "I need to ask: Do you like it when I do that? Is there something you'd like better?"

5. **Oral sex—or the lack thereof.** "I love this and want more!" or "I don't enjoy doing this. Is it okay if I pleasure you in a different way instead?"

6. **Anal sex.** "Are you ready to go there with me?"

7. **Porn.** "You know I like porn. How about if we share it for a change, and see what transpires?" or "Let's 'shop' for new ideas in these magazines."

8. **Dress up.** "It would drive me crazy if you'd wear something like *this!*"

9. **Opening it up.** "I'd like to try a threesome. I'd like to open up our relationship to the possibility of involving other lovers. Are you interested in that?"

10. **Same sex.** "I never told you this, but I've always wondered what it would be like with another woman. Want to help me answer that question? Would you mind if I explored this on my own?"

11. **Dark side.** "I'd like to indulge my fantasies." "There's something I dream about that I've never told you." "Let's go shopping for toys!" "Let's learn some new games!" "Let's do it in a new place!" "What are *your* fantasies?"

You get the idea. I'm sure you have lots on your mind that you'd like to share with your lover as a prelude to new and wonderful sexual experiences. Take that leap of faith by opening up the conversation, and, oh, the places you'll go!

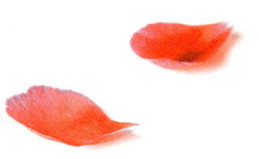

Let's Talk Dirty!

As I said, talk is a two-part subject. In addition to becoming comfortable with talking *about* sex, you might want to add some sexy talk to your repertoire. Talk really can be the *other* oral sex once you get used to the idea, and you might be surprised at what a turn-on it is. Whether you are directing, describing, responding, or just emoting, adding the verbal dimension to your sensual experience can make the two of you feel more in tune and in the moment. It might even make you feel like a couple of porn stars!

What Do You Call It?

The first challenge in sex talk is getting comfortable with the words themselves. You might have to overcome some of those good manners you learned, that little voice in your head that tells you that certain words aren't polite or nice or proper. Time to cut loose—and in order to do that, you might even want to rehearse out loud when you are alone. The more comfortable you can get with the language of explicit sex, the more fun you'll have when you are with your partner.

Do you call it a *cock* or a *dick*? A *cunt* or a *pussy* or a *slit*? *Tits* or *boobs* or *breasts*? These little words might make you snicker at first, but they can be powerful aphrodisiacs for both of you when used in the heat of the moment. With some experimentation (alone and together), you'll find the words that really communicate for you—and turn you both on. As an exercise, try saying some of these sentences aloud until you feel completely comfortable. Choose the ones that fit your gender and preferences, of course—and put some passion into it!

Your pussy looks so sweet and delicious—I can't wait to taste those juices!

Let me get my hands on that big, burning cock!

I want to feel your mouth all over me. Suck on my breasts until I scream!

Split me open while I ride you like a bull!

Squeeze me with your sweet, tight cunt!

Suck it harder! Suck it 'til I come!

I love feeling your tongue deep inside my naughty slit!

You might feel silly at first if you aren't used to talking like this, but you'll get used to it and will soon want to try it out on your lover. Now come up with some choice phrases of your own, using your lover's best attributes and burning desires for inspiration. Practice, practice, practice—and then unleash it on your mate the next time you have a golden opportunity.

It may seem as if we've strayed from the topic of foreplay here, but adding the dimension of language to your sexual play takes a little preparation, and preparation is what foreplay is all about. Learn to talk the talk and you can put it into play when the time comes. And this is one area where your mate is bound to match you point for point. Talk inspires talk. Soon, you'll both be using lusty language before as well as during sex, and driving each other wild in the process.

Language of Love

In a long-term relationship, using very specific, personal language in lovemaking can deepen your bond and enhance your intimacy as a couple. Once you've become comfortable with dirty talk, you will find yourselves developing and refining your own private bedroom language, including special terms of endearment; shorthand ways of expressing what you want, what you like, and what you need in the heat of the moment; and even special names for your favorite activities and for each other's sex organs and moves.

Some couples love to call each other *bastard* and *bitch* during sex, finding that a little bit of verbal aggression or abuse makes it all the more passionate (and all is forgiven later). Others melt into ecstasy with the help of terms such as *loverboy*, *sweet baby*, and *darling one*.

If you want to get your man pumped up like never before, come up with ways to praise his massive and masterful endowment: Terms such as *big man*, *poppa*, *cocksman*, and *swordsman* will make him stand at attention. Likewise, guys, try *sugarpussy*, *sweet slit*, *tight lips*, and the like. There's no such thing as a word that is too nasty, too silly, or too explicit if it turns you both on. Once you've got the vocabulary, you can make sure you both get what you need as never before.

Using Your Words

There are a few specific ways that you can incorporate talk into your routine. The language of love (or lust) can help you:

Describe what you are doing to your lover, or planning to do, in salacious detail. "I'm going to lick those nipples until they are hard and begging for more!" "Can you feel my hard cock deep inside you?"

Direct and encourage your lover. "Give it to me harder!" "Don't stop licking me—faster, faster!"

Respond to what your lover is doing. "God, that feels so good—I'm going to come all over you!"

Emote using sounds as well as words—sighs, grunts, screams, whatever expresses all that you feel. "Ohmigod, yes! OOOhhhh, that's incredible! Don't stop!"

Breathe. Using words and sounds actually helps you breathe more deeply and rhythmically, which will enhance your sensations and, ultimately, your orgasm(s). Every word or sound you make involves an exhalation, every gasp an inhalation. Exercising your lungs and diaphragm, propelling oxygen in and out of your body, will fuel you more fully—all the way to the point of peak pleasure. (And those gasps, moans, and instructions will inspire your lover to come right along with you!)

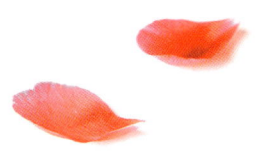

Sex Talk as a Prelude

One last thing about "the other oral sex." It really can be used as foreplay, especially when you take advantage of today's technology. Phone sex may have been around since just after Mr. Bell perfected the device, but nowadays we carry our phones everywhere, making any street corner a potential venue for some dirty talk. (And taking that palm-sized cell to bed with you for a late-night session with a long-distance lover is a lot easier than trying to wield the old corded model with the monster receiver.)

How long do you think it took somebody to turn texting into sexting? Not long, I bet—and then along came Skype and iChat and the like, so now we can indulge in visuals as well as words, giving a whole new meaning to the question "Get the picture?"

By all means, think about adding phone and cybersex sessions to your foreplay routine:

Use a phone call, voicemail message, e-mail, or text to tell your lover what—exactly—you are thinking about as you anticipate your evening together.

Text your lover briefly throughout the day, reminding her that there are only five more hours, four more hours, three more hours, etc., until you will ravish her luscious body. (Don't forget the details!)

Leave an old-fashioned "heavy breathing" message incorporating the best impression of the sounds you two make when in the throes of great sex to get his blood pumping and his mind racing.

Share a sexy private phone-sex (or Skype) session where you direct each other to touch yourselves in specifically delicious ways, culminating in shared orgasms and sweet aftertalk. If you are a Skyper, doff those clothes and let your lover see what you're talking about!

The Love Questionnaire

Here's another way to communicate your fantasies, desires, questions, and notions to your lover—and learn more about him or her in return. It's a very nice little exercise, too, especially if you've ever wanted to try your hand at writing frankly about sex.

This private exchange takes place on paper rather than in real time. Make two copies of the following questions (plus any others you might want to add), one for each of you. Then go off on your own, take your time, and answer each question as honestly and completely as you can. (You can use the computer to type your answers or handwrite them.) When you're done, put your responses into an envelope with your lover's name on it and leave them under her pillow, in his briefcase or sock drawer—anywhere that is completely private.

Once you've read each other's answers, you can discuss them—or not. That's completely up to you. Sometimes it's nice to just skip the conversation and start putting what you've learned about each other into practice, working together to live out your fantasies, improve your sex lives, and explore new pathways to pleasure. Here are some questions to get you started; by all means, feel free to add others that are relevant to the two of you.

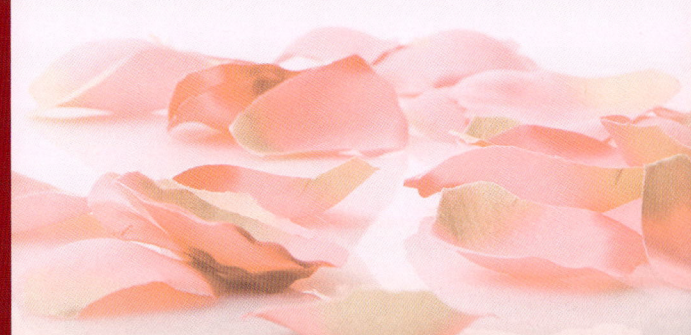

1. These are the things I find most beautiful, striking, and sexy about you.

_____

2. My favorite thing about our sex life is

_____ .

3. Here's something you do to me/we do together that I wish you'd/we'd do more often.

_____

4. Here's something you/we do that I don't really enjoy.

_____

5. There are some things we've never tried. I'd very much like to

_____ .

6. There are some questions I've never had the nerve to ask you. Here they are!

_____

7. We all have fantasies, and I want to share my deepest ones with you, starting with this one.

_____

8. I know there are things about me that you want to know. Here are some very personal things I haven't yet shared with you.

_____

CHAPTER 10

AFTERPLAY

Although this book is designed to focus on the preliminaries, it wouldn't seem right to end without a few words about the sweet afterglow of great sex—your reward as a couple for coming together with great passion and a commitment to mutual satisfaction. If foreplay is about paving the way to memorable sex, afterplay is about cementing the bond you've created and expanding the closeness and feelings of love that great sex inspires.

Afterplay provides a sense of fulfillment and completion and helps you carry that emotional high into other aspects of your life together. As with foreplay, it's important not to rush through the period that follows orgasm—and why would you want to? You've just shared a peak physical and emotional experience. It's time to linger in the moment, stroke, breathe, sigh, talk, laugh . . . and luxuriate.

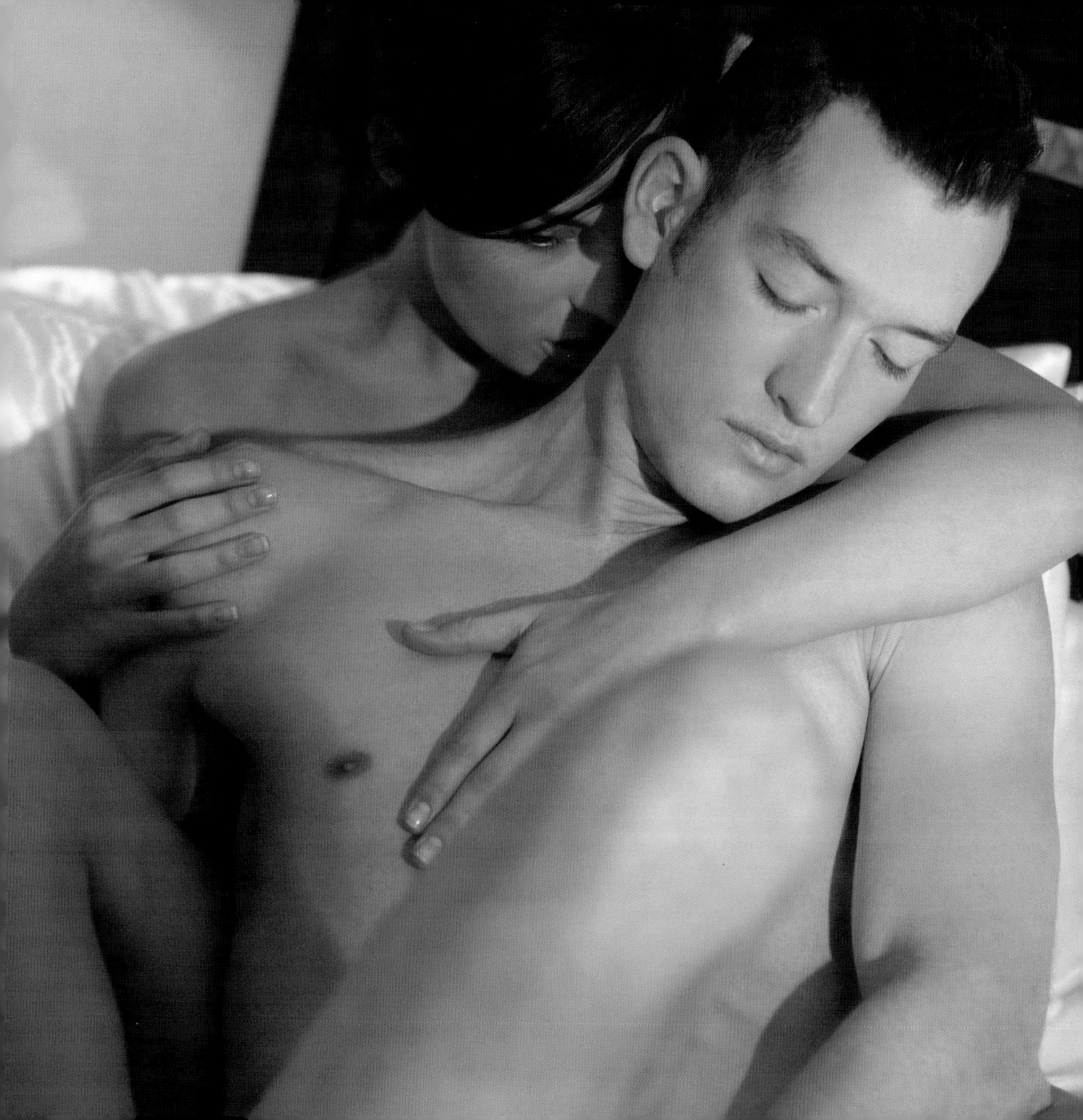

The Science Side

Chemically, you've each released specific hormones—which accounts for some of the differences in how you feel. Following intercourse, the male brain tends to retreat to a rest state, leaving him drained and sleepy; his heartbeat and body temperature are dropping even as his penis is shrinking to its "everyday" size. A woman's brain, on the other hand, is stimulated after orgasm, leaving her alert and with a desire to bond. Just as it takes a woman longer, in general, to become aroused, it takes her longer to come down from the heights of sexual pleasure. This difference doesn't have to create a conflict, though. With an awareness of the situation, you can indulge each other's natural tendencies, compromise, and enjoy the afterglow in harmony. Ladies, don't be stunned or hurt if your man zones out or even dozes off after sex—it is natural and usually temporary. Guys, understand that your lover's urge to cuddle and coo is motivated in part by her chemistry—and what's so bad about some postcoital cuddling?

Keep It Simple and Gentle

As I said, it can be a nice time to talk, but avoid turning afterplay into a postmortem of what preceded it. Beyond a few appreciative comments about what you've just accomplished, leave any critiques of your sexual performance for a later time and different place. (See chapter 9 for more on the subject of sex talk.) Laughter, on the other hand, makes for great afterplay. Sex can get very intense and dramatic—which is delightful—but afterward, it can be nice to lighten the mood, share a joke, or just be silly together.

There are many kinds of touch, as discussed throughout this book, but for afterplay the gentlest touch is best. All of your senses have been heightened, so a deep massage or a nipple-tweak might not be the best move. Stick with gentle caresses: light, all-over kisses; nuzzling; lying forehead to forehead or cheek to cheek; a soft earlobe suck—subtle, comforting things that feel great as your blood is redistributing itself all over your body.

Round Two?

Sometimes, attentive and satisfying afterplay can lead to . . . more sex! Don't be surprised if you are both ready to go again after an hour or so. I know—you won't always have the time to devote to multiple rounds of magical sex. But once in a while, try setting aside a whole afternoon to enjoy each other. Have some snacks and beverages ready to replenish your resources, your favorite bathrobes to keep you cozy, and the Sunday paper to read together or a favorite movie on DVD to dip into while you're waiting for the urge to return. Chat, kiss, caress, and . . . who knows what might raise its beautiful head again?

The Beginning

I love the idea of ending this book with a section called "The Beginning"—because I hope that reading and using it will mark the beginning of a fabulous new sex life for you and your partner, filled with sensual highs, mutual satisfaction, and deepening intimacy. Beginnings are so important, and great foreplay is the sweetest beginning of all—opening the door to all that you desire in the bedroom and beyond.

Enjoy!

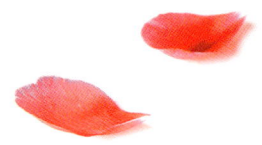

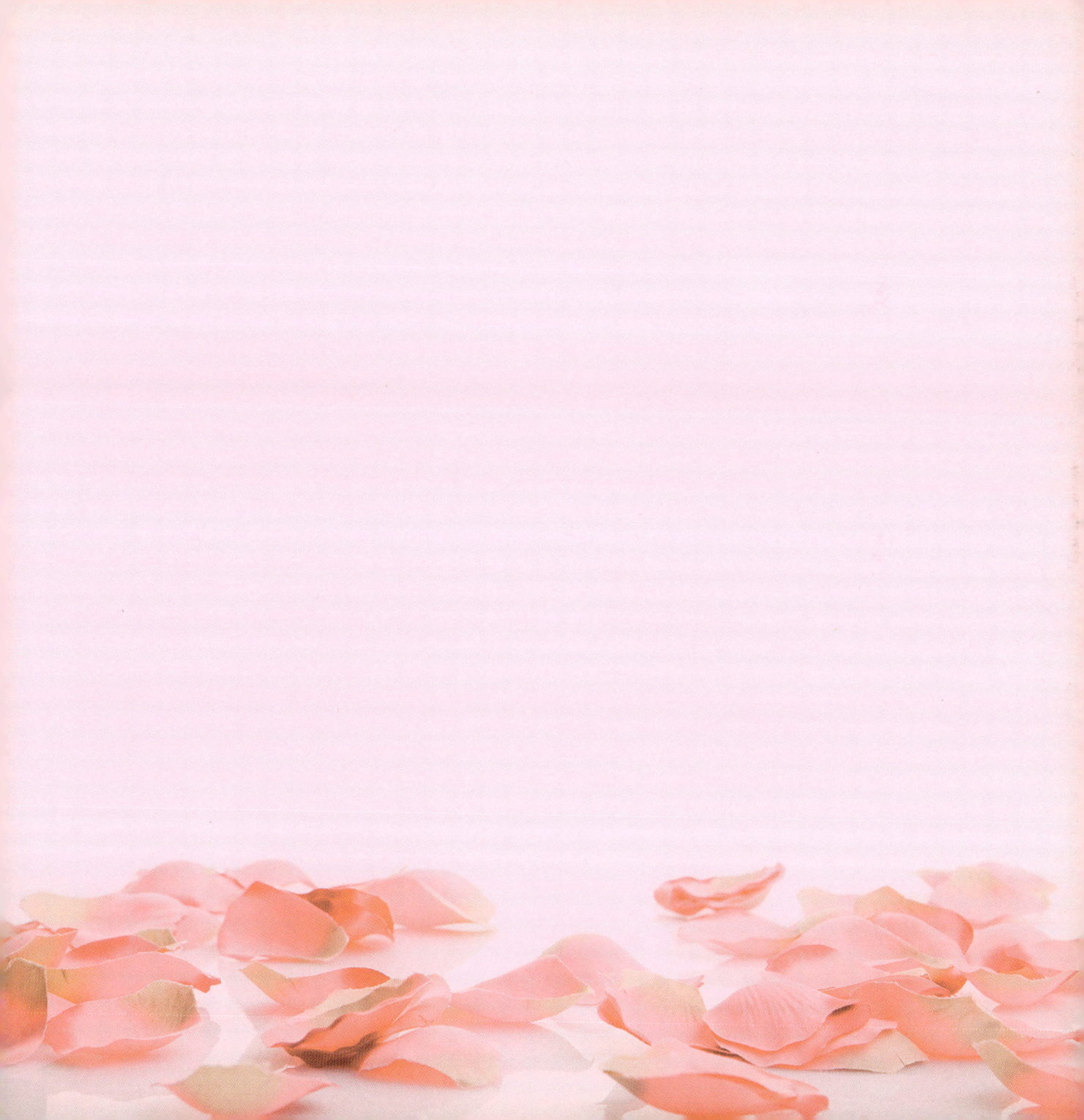

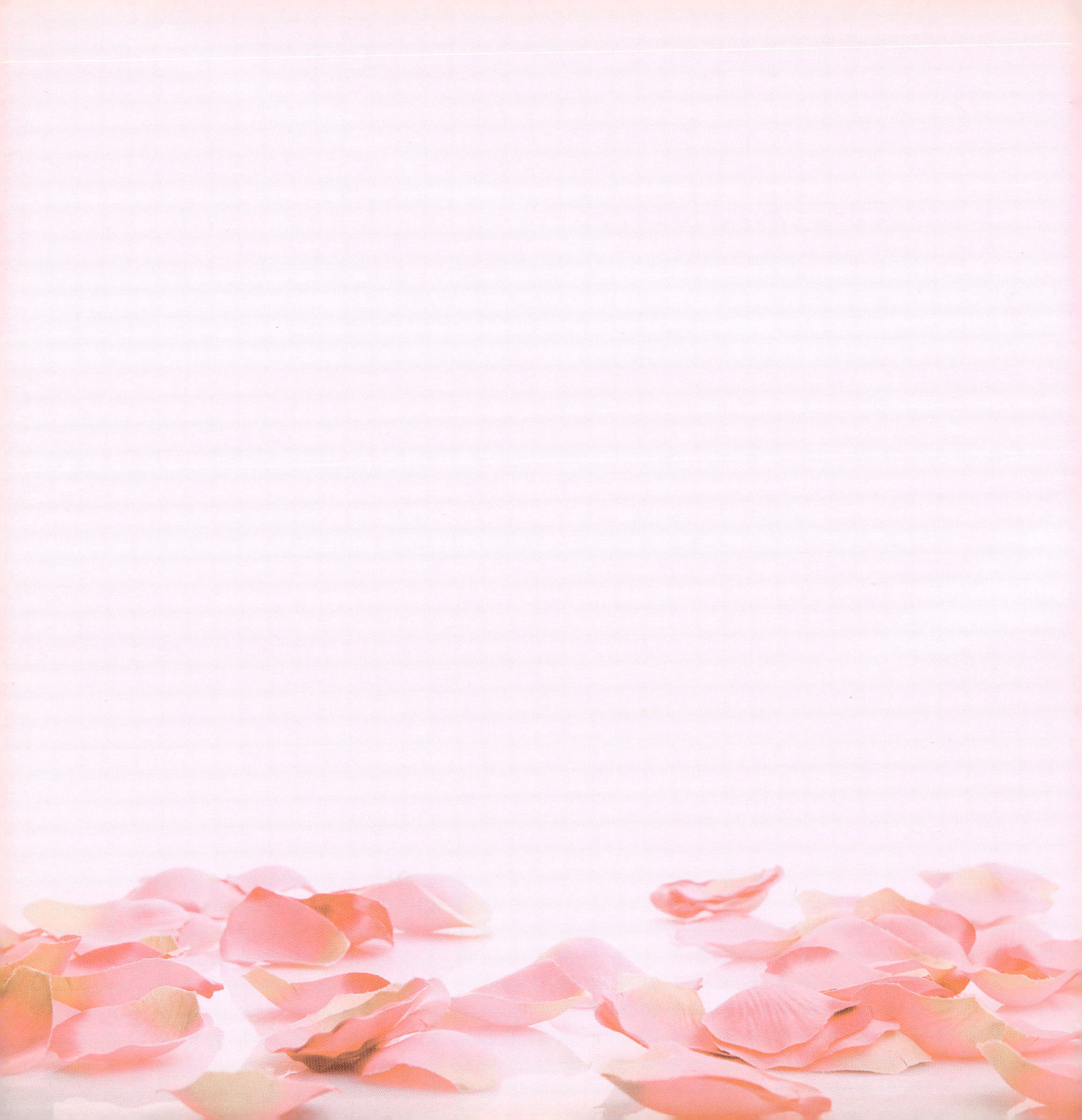

Acknowledgments

For their foresight, forethought, and forbearance, the author would like to thank Will Kiester, Jill Alexander, Anne Bobby, Barbara Call, Leslie Ben-Zvi, Steve Gettinger, John Gettings.

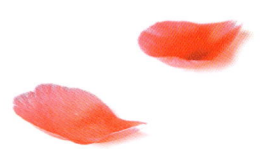